T0251634

*Routledge Revivals*

# Social Work in Child Care

In the late 1960s the child care service had undergone considerable change, and was to change again after the Seebohm Committee had reported. Yet its central tasks had become clear: preventive work; the reception of children into care, work with them and their parents during the period of care; the selection of foster parents; work with foster parents, and with residential staff; and adoption.

Originally published in 1968, the present work devotes a chapter to each of these important tasks, and examines the role of the child care staff within the local authority department at the time, though many of the arguments of the book will also be applicable to the work of the voluntary child care organisations of the day.

# Social Work in Child Care

### Elisabeth Pugh

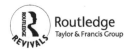
Routledge
Taylor & Francis Group

First published in 1968
by Routledge & Kegan Paul Ltd

This edition first published in 2023 by Routledge
4 Park Square, Milton Park, Abingdon, Oxon, OX14 4RN

and by Routledge
605 Third Avenue, New York, NY 10017

*Routledge is an imprint of the Taylor & Francis Group, an informa business*

**Publisher's Note**
The publisher has gone to great lengths to ensure the quality of this reprint but points out that some imperfections in the original copies may be apparent.

**Disclaimer**
The publisher has made every effort to trace copyright holders and welcomes correspondence from those they have been unable to contact.

A Library of Congress record exists under ISBN: 071006148X

ISBN: 978-1-032-44069-9 (hbk)
ISBN: 978-1-003-37030-7 (ebk)
ISBN: 978-1-032-44077-4 (pbk)

Book DOI 10.4324/9781003370307

# Social Work in Child Care

*by Elisabeth Pugh*

*Formerly Deputy Children's Officer, Somerset County Council*

**LONDON**

**ROUTLEDGE & KEGAN PAUL**

**NEW YORK: HUMANITIES PRESS**

First Published 1968
by Routledge & Kegan Paul Ltd
Broadway House, 68-74 Carter Lane
London, E.C.4

Printed in Great Britain
by Garden City Press Ltd
Letchworth, Hertfordshire

SBN 7100 6148 x (C)
SBN 7100 6149 8 (P)

# General editor's introduction

THE LIBRARY OF SOCIAL WORK is designed to meet the needs of students following courses of training for social work. In recent years the number and kinds of training in Britain have increased in an unprecedented way. But there has been no corresponding increase in the supply of text-books to cover the growing differentiation of subject matter or to respond to the growing spirit of enthusiastic but critical enquiry into the range of subjects relevant to social work. The Library will consist of short texts designed to introduce the student to the main features of each topic of enquiry, to the significant theoretical contributions so far made to its understanding, and to some of the outstanding problems. Each volume will suggest ways in which the student might continue his work by further reading.

The child care service, as Elisabeth Pugh illustrates, has undergone considerable change in recent years, and it is likely to change again after the Seebohm Committee has reported. Yet its central tasks have become clear: preventive work; the reception of children into care, work with them and their parents during the period of care; the selection of foster parents; work with foster parents, and with residential staff; and adoption.

These tasks must be performed within an administrative structure that facilitates performance and enables all concerned to deepen their knowledge. The author devotes a chapter to each of these important tasks, and finally examines the role of the child care staff within the local authority department.

This book is one of a series devoted to an exploration of the different branches into which social work is at present commonly divided. Its focus is the child care service of the local authority, but much of its argument will be applicable to the work of the voluntary child care organisations. The book is based on the conviction that the child care officer is both caseworker and local government official (or presumably the officer of a voluntary organisation), and that 'there is no point at which ceasing to be concerned with administration, she becomes exclusively a caseworker'. The author, therefore, takes time to examine the legal and adminstrative framework of the work, but this is not done at the expense of a careful differentiation of the tasks of the worker including their psychological aspects.

NOEL TIMMS

# Contents

# 1

# Introduction and history

## Introduction

This book presents an outline of the work of a local authority children's department from the standpoint of a social worker in this setting. The child care officer is both caseworker and local government officer: she is concerned to meet the needs of individuals and of families within a defined legal and administrative framework. The law defines her duties and powers; the administrative setting provides and limits her resources; and her casework skills determine the way in which she uses herself and these resources in relation to clients. There is no point at which, ceasing to be concerned with administration, she becomes exclusively a caseworker; no point at which she is concerned with the legal aspects of a case and not with the needs of those involved in it. Law, administration and casework are the three dimensions of child care. For this reason every chapter in the book contains some consideration of each. An overall view of this kind necessitates many omissions, but further reading is suggested in Chapter 9.

In order to simplify a complicated subject, the legal and administrative framework described in these pages is that of a local authority children's department. The very considerable contribution to child care provision made in this country by voluntary agencies must not for this reason be overlooked. In 1966, out of some 80,000 children in care in England and Wales, about 13% were in the care of voluntary children's societies; 96 out of 126 approved schools are provided by voluntary agencies; voluntary bodies, the pioneers of adoption work, are still responsible for a large proportion of placements each year; the Family Service Units, Family Welfare Association and other non-statutory agencies were concerned with family care well before children's departments came into being, and local authorities owe much to the skills and methods they evolved. Much of this book is relevant to the work of non-statutory bodies because many of them are engaged in similar and related areas of work and are to some extent affected by the same legislation as the local government children's department.

In the next chapter reference is made to the appointment by the Government of a committee with Mr. Frederick Seebohm as chairman to review the organisation of local authority personal social services. Whatever changes may take place in the light of the recommendations of this committee or, indeed, in the general structure of local government, the necessity for any future social work service to be concerned with the needs of children will continue undiminished.

Two other general points should be made at this stage. In order to avoid confusion child care officers are allotted the pronouns 'she' and 'her' and individual children are referred to as 'he' and 'him'. The only justification for this is clarity in presentation. Secondly, in connection with juvenile court proceedings a child is legally defined as a person under the age of fourteen years, and a young person as one who has attained the age of fourteen years and is under the age of seventeen years. For convenience, in this book the words 'child' or 'children' will include young person(s) unless otherwise stated.

## Historical background

The Children Act of 1948, which created children's committees, was part of the legislation which marked the end of the Poor Law in this country. Public authorities had had some statutory responsibilities for destitute children since a series of Acts of Parliament in the sixteenth century. This legislation was codified in the Elizabethan Poor Relief Act of 1601, which gave church wardens and parish overseers the power to levy rates and to set to work or bind as apprentices vagrant and pauper children. Those who could not work were accommodated with adult paupers in workhouses. In the nineteenth century the parishes were grouped into larger units known as poor law unions, each with an elected Board of Guardians of the Poor. These unions continued until the Local Government Act of 1929 made the provision of poor relief the responsibility of county and county borough councils. But by 1948, when children's departments were set up, local authorities were not only concerned with the care of poor children. During the latter part of the nineteenth and the first half of the twentieth century their statutory duties had extended to cover some aspects of the care of children who were delinquent, cruelly treated, neglected, or living with private foster mothers. They exercised these responsibilities not through their public assistance committees dealing with destitute children, but through their education and health commit-

3

tees. There were, thus, by 1948 at least three local government departments concerned with the care of children away from home.

Local authorities were not, of course, the only bodies providing for children. During the eighteenth and nineteenth centuries a succession of philanthropists and reformers, inspired by religious and humanitarian ideals, had tried to stir the national conscience about children in need of care. Among others were Thomas Coram, the retired sea captain who started the Foundling Hospital; Mary Carpenter who established the first reformatory school for delinquents; Dr. Barnardo; Stephenson of the National Children's Home; Edward Rudolf of the Waifs and Strays; Cardinal Vaughan of the Crusade of Rescue. These were pioneers who not only themselves made provision for homeless, neglected or delinquent children, but also by their example influenced for good the methods of care employed by the poor law authorities.

The mass evacuation of children from large towns during the second world war made the general public aware of the poverty and squalor in which many families were living. It also drew attention to the needs of children away from home. In the climate of social change and reform at the end of the war, concern was expressed not only about slum conditions in the cities, but also about the inadequacy and poor quality of the provision made for children in public care.

These widespread feelings of concern were brought into focus by the death in January 1945, of a twelve-year-old foster child, Dennis O'Neill. This boy, committed to the care of a local authority on the grounds of his parents' cruelty, was found at the inquest to have been neglected and cruelly treated by foster parents living in another area. The public enquiry which followed revealed a lack of supervision, which was partly the result of administrative confusion between the local authorities concerned. Before the report of the enquiry had been published the Government had set up, as a matter of urgency, a departmental committee under the chairmanship of Miss Myra Curtis. Their duties were 'to enquire into existing methods of providing for children who from loss of parents or from any cause whatever are deprived of a normal home life with their own parents or relatives; and to consider what further measures should be taken to ensure that these children are brought up under conditions best calculated to compensate them for the lack of parental care'. The widespread use of the words 'deprived children' springs from these terms of reference of the Curtis Committee.

The Committee's report (1946) enumerated the many different local and central government departments concerned with the care of deprived children and drew attention to the consequent administrative muddle. It also depicted in vivid detail the variety of provision then available for children living away from home. Although legislation had attempted to curtail the use of workhouses for children, there were still young children accommodated in these institutions with old, infirm and mentally disordered adults. Other children were in special homes built in the workhouse grounds; in large institutions holding upwards of two hundred children; in self-contained groups of small cottage homes; in scattered homes on housing estates; in residential nurseries; and a minority of children were boarded out in foster homes. Although there was considerable variety in both the methods and standards of provision for deprived children, the Committee was not satisfied with the overall quality of care provided, and made a number of recommendations. The first was that a Central Training Council in Child Care should be set up to promote training courses for residential and field staff and to recruit staff of high quality to the service.

But a trained residential and field staff would not be enough. The administrative framework needed strengthening and simplifying. The main recommendations of the Curtis Committee in this respect were embodied in the 1948 Children Act.

## The Children Act 1948

This Act, which laid the foundations of our existing child care services, provides that every county and county borough council should establish a children's committee and appoint a children's officer. The new committees took over the children who were the responsibility of the local authority under the Poor Law Act, which was repealed, and were given the duty of receiving into care those children whose parents were unable or unfit to care for them. They were also given responsibility for functions carried out by other committees of the local authority under previous legislation: the supervision of private foster children and children placed for adoption, the care of children committed to the authority by a juvenile court, the registration of adoption societies, the provision of approved school and remand home accommodation. At central government level, the Home Office became the responsible department.

As the Curtis Committee recommended, the children's committee was to be the sole local government body responsible for all deprived children in their area. The Act explicitly states the duty of the committee towards the

6

child in their care: 'to exercise their powers with respect to him so as to further his best interests, and to afford him opportunity for the proper development of his character and abilities'. Children in care were seen not as paupers or criminals, but as individuals with needs and potentialities which the new committees must help to fulfil.

Children's officers and their staff were at first almost entirely occupied in providing accommodation for the children they had inherited from other departments, and for the increasing numbers who came into care every year: during the first four years of the life of the new departments, the numbers of children in care over the whole country rose dramatically by about 21,000. The rising costs of the new service led the Select Committee on Estimates in 1951–52 to recommend that local authorities should direct their attention towards preventing the domestic upheaval and distress that resulted in children having to leave home.

Financial considerations, however, were only one of several factors which during the 1950s, led children's departments to consider the problems of the child's own family. John Bowlby's monograph (1951) reviewed existing studies of children separated from their mothers at an early age, and drew attention to the personality disturbance that can result from this experience. This book had considerable impact on child care practice in this country, partly because the research findings it described were mirrored in the day-to-day experience of children's officers and their staff. It became apparent that the greatly improved material conditions now provided by children's committees were not in themselves sufficient to create the environment in which children in care could grow into emotionally mature adults. The increased numbers of

7

better trained staff led to a clearer perception of the needs of individual children in homes and nurseries, and revealed an alarming proportion of the apparently affectionless personalities described by Bowlby.

During their first twelve years the new children's departments experimented with various kinds of provision for children in an attempt to prevent the evils of institutionalisation. The development of what would now be regarded as indiscriminate boarding out, resulted in a high rate of damaging foster home breakdowns. Many authorities replaced their large homes with small family group homes accommodating no more than ten children. Although these were successful in some areas and for some children, it soon became apparent that substitute families could not be created by this means, and that they could offer little more security in personal relationships than the average foster home. Children's departments were gradually led to the conclusion that for most children substitute care could only be a second best, and that more attention must be paid to keeping children in their own homes. Moreover, the children themselves led child care staff to consider their parents. More time could now be given to talking with children in care about their ideas and feelings, and many revealed a deep sense of loss, and a longing to know more about their background, which had previously been camouflaged by a superficial unconcern.

The 1948 Children Act had for the first time given local authorities the duty to restore children to their parents if this was consistent with the welfare of the child. For children who had been in care of public assistance authorities for many years, this often proved impossible. Some parents were completely untraceable: others had become resigned to the absence of their children and had lost the impetus to re-establish their family life. It was clearly necessary to maintain contact with parents and to work with them throughout the period their child spent in care if restoration was to be successful.

The aim of most of the enlightened work of the child care pioneers and their successors had been to rescue children from bad and damaging home environments, and by the provision of favourable conditions and instruction to save their souls and prevent the development of a criminal character. The experience of children's departments in their first few years led them to look at the parents themselves, to seek to understand the circumstances which caused the disruption or break-up of family life, and to develop the necessary casework skills to help parents and children in their own homes. Family casework was increasingly emphasised and came to be regarded as an integral part of the work of the department. The change in name of the field work staff from Boarding Out Officers to Child Care Officers, and in some instances to Family Caseworkers, was a minor indication of this change in outlook. Section 1 of the Children and Young Persons Act of 1963, which is discussed in the next chapter, gave statutory authority to these new developments in the work.

# 2
# Working with parents and children at home

## Background

The end of the last chapter described how the needs of children in care led child care staff into working with their parents. The development of family casework by children's departments has, however, sprung also from a concern for children in their own homes who are neglected, ill-treated or beyond parental control. In 1948, very shortly before children's departments came into being, the Women's Group on Public Welfare issued a report on their enquiry into the problems of these children. The report recommended:

(i) that there should be greater co-ordination of work among social agencies dealing with neglected children;

(ii) that the local authority should be clearly responsible for seeing that any necessary prosecutions are instituted in these cases; and

(iii) that local authorities should provide an extended, specialised, family casework service.

*Co-ordination of work with families*

In July 1950, following a parliamentary debate, a circular was issued to county and county borough councils by the Home Office, the Ministry of Health and the Ministry of Education. This joint circular recommended that councils should designate one of their officers as having a special responsibility for co-ordinating the work of statutory and voluntary agencies concerned with the welfare of children in their own homes. The officer so designated, in some authorities the children's officer, in others the medical officer of health, education officer or clerk, is responsible for holding regular meetings at which the needs of neglected or cruelly treated children are considered. The co-ordinating officer may also arrange case conferences at which the social workers involved in a particular family situation may discuss the direction of their work and try to agree on any necessary action.

There is some disagreement about the measure of success which may be claimed by the co-ordinating machinery described above. *Co-ordination Reviewed* (Stevenson, 1963) illustrates some of the difficulties involved when a group of people with different functions, attitudes and training meet to discuss a multi-problem family. The workers concerned are employed by various agencies with differing and even conflicting objectives; it is unlikely, however, that the problems of co-ordinating would automatically disappear with any future merging of different departments into a family service. Co-ordinating meetings and case conferences have at least helped the different social work agencies to see intercommunication and co-operation as a worthy aim. Further, they may even have had some part in reducing the horde of workers who, it was once alleged, swooped avidly on each and every family with multiple problems.

## Action in cases of neglect and ill-treatment

In 1948 the powers and duties of children's departments to help children in their own homes were limited to those provided by the Children and Young Persons Act of 1933. Section 62 which, slightly amended, is still in force gives local authorities the duty to bring before a juvenile court 'any child or young person residing or found in their district' who appears to them to be in need of care, protection or control 'unless they are satisfied that the taking of proceedings is undesirable in his interests or that proceedings are about to be taken by some other person'. Section 2 of the Children and Young Persons (Amendment) Act 1952 gives authorities the further duty of causing enquiries to be made if they receive information that a child or young person is in need of care or protection, unless they are satisfied that such enquiries are unnecessary.

Children's departments thus have the clear duty of protecting the child in his own home by enquiry into allegations of neglect and cruel treatment, and if necessary by appropriate legal action. This may include application to a magistrate for an order on which a child may in an emergency be removed from his parents and taken to a 'place of safety'.

These provisions introduce an unmistakable element of authority into a child care officer's work with families in their own homes. The power to take children away, albeit only with the consent of a magistrate, is considered by some workers to be so threatening in its implications that it cannot be carried by those who are engaged in family casework. Further reference will be made to this problem in the concluding section of this chapter.

### A family casework service

The third recommendation of the Women's Group on Public Welfare in 1948 was that local authorities should set up an extended, specialised, family casework service. Eight years later the Ingleby Committee had among its terms of reference the powers and duties of local authorities to prevent or forestall the suffering of children through neglect in their own homes. The duty to locate and deal with neglect or ill-treatment was not enough: it was necessary to devise means of preventing its occurrence. The Ingleby Committee recommended that these duties should be given to local authorities, together with the power to carry out preventive casework and meet the material needs of families if necessary. The Committee's report emphasises the importance of early detection of families at risk and commends the idea of a unified family service to the Government for further study. A Committee under the chairmanship of Mr. Frederick Seebohm is currently reviewing the organisation of the local authority personal social services and considering what changes are desirable to secure an effective family service.

### The Children and Young Persons Act 1963

In the meantime, however, some of the recommendations of the Ingleby Committee were given effect in the Children and Young Persons Act of 1963. Section 1 of this Act lays a duty on local authorities 'to make available such advice, guidance and assistance as may promote the welfare of children by diminishing the need to receive children into or keep them in care . . . or to bring children before a juvenile court; and any provisions made by a local authority under this sub-section may, if the local authority think fit, include provision for giving assistance in kind, or in exceptional circumstances in cash.'

The section continues by authorising local authorities to make arrangements with voluntary organisations to carry out this work on their behalf.

These provisions are historic in that for the first time the councils of counties and county boroughs are specifically empowered to spend money on keeping families together. Legal authority was thereby given to the long-term preventive work that many of them had been carrying out for some time in order to lessen the neglect and ill-treatment of children in their own homes and to avoid unnecessary reception into care. The duty to work to diminish the need to bring children before a juvenile court gives local authorities new responsibilities for the prevention of delinquency. Delinquency, child neglect, ill-treatment and reception into care are for the first time in law brought together as indications of the danger of family breakdown.

Moreover, for the first time public authorities are in this section empowered to give money, not on the basis of strict equality but according to need. Pensions and social security benefits are all calculated on scales which are designed to ensure the demonstrable fairness which comes from giving people in similar circumstances exactly equal amounts of money. Implicit in section 1 of the 1963 Act is both the realisation that individual families in need may find themselves in circumstances not covered by the normal benefits; and also the acknowledgment that some people are so prevented by social or mental inadequacy from using their incomes in a wise and prudent way that additional assistance is necessary. There is in fact the implied recognition that true fairness does not consist in exact equality of treatment but must relate to individual capacity and need. All sections of the community do not of course accept this principle and children's officers in exercising their power under the first part of the 1963 Act have had to have some regard for public opinion.

It should here be noted that although the functions of the local authority under section 1 of the Act stand referred specifically to the children's committee, local authorities may—and in fact occasionally do—give their welfare or health committees power to spend money under this section.

Local authorities have used their powers under section 1 of the Children and Young Persons Act in a variety of ways. Specialist casework staff have been appointed in many areas to work with children and families in their own homes; family advice centres have been set up and publicised; a few residential centres for families who are homeless or in need of intensive help have been established; some authorities have experimented with special clubs and play centres for the children of socially handicapped parents. There has been an increasing realisation of the importance of encouraging early notification of families at risk, not only by social caseworkers, education welfare officers, teachers and health visitors, but also by housing managers, county court officials who are aware of proceedings for debt, building societies contemplating foreclosing on mortgages, family doctors, ministers of religion, gas and electricity boards likely to cut off supplies. In many authorities the police consult with the staff of the children's department before bringing children before a juvenile court. In an attempt to prevent unnecessary admissions to care because of short-term illness or confinement, a few authorities have developed schemes of daily care—either by special domiciliary workers or by a panel of approved daily minders: at least one rural authority maintains a fleet of dormobiles in which full-time women workers may live while they are caring for a family in the mother's absence. There has, however, been a greater acknowledgment by children's departments that some short-term admissions to care can in themselves be 'preventive' if they are used to reduce tensions which might otherwise have brought a family to breaking point.

Help has been given with clothes, furniture and household equipment, materials for home decoration, and fares to enable relatives to travel to look after children who would otherwise have to be received into care. Payments have been made outright or on a loan basis to reconnect gas and electricity supplies, to complete the down payment on a caravan or the first month's rent in advance, and guarantees against loss of rent have been given to housing authorities.

This outline of ways in which authorities have used their powers under section 1 of the Children and Young Persons Act is not intended to be exhaustive, nor to give the impression that all children's departments are providing some or indeed any of these facilities. The development of services for families has in fact been very patchy. In some authorities little progress has been made in this direction— in others, work with families has become the responsibility of the health, welfare or education departments, and the children's department confines itself to its statutory duties in connection with neglected or ill-treated children and to prevention at the stage when an application for care has been made. There are authorities, however, where the children's department is attempting to provide a comprehensive family casework service, and in some instances its name has in fact been altered to the Family Care Department.

Mention must be made of one other legal provision relating to the duty of the local authority towards children in their own homes. Section 3 of the 1963 Children and Young Persons Act deprives a parent of the right to bring his child before a juvenile court on the grounds that he is unable to control him. Instead, the parent must request the local authority to bring the child before the appropriate court on the grounds that he is in need of care, protection or control. If the local authority refuses to do so, or fails to do so within twenty-eight days from the date the notice is given, the parent may appeal to a juvenile court for an order, directing the local authority to take this action. In practice this section means that parents are prevented from acting precipitately and that children's departments are given the opportunity to offer casework help on a voluntary basis. In many instances the drastic step of exposing, and thereby exacerbating, the conflict between parent and child in court can be avoided. Much of the work with children and parents under this section is, of course, with adolescents. Here the residential facilities of the children's department can provide an opportunity for lowering tensions by the temporary removal of the young person from an emotionally untenable situation.

*Family casework in a local authority setting*

As we have seen, work with families has developed out of efforts to find alternatives to reception into care, out of the need to rehabilitate children already in care, and out of the duty to identify and protect the neglected, cruelly treated child. Children's departments have moved from a narrow concept of preventive work, first-aid at the point of crisis, to some attempt to provide a service for families. The need for a service of this kind became evident with the increasing awareness among child care workers that problems such as homelessness, and the rejection, ill-treatment or neglect of children should not be treated in isolation but as symptoms of family malfunctioning, and as ways in which the stresses within the life of the family, or between the family and the community, find expression. There have, of course, been similar developments in other settings: delinquency, criminality, mental illness and various forms of physical ill-health in one member of a family have been observed as reflections of complex processes of interaction within the family as a whole.

This present tendency among social workers to see the family as the unit of casework treatment is of course rooted in psychoanalytic concepts of the importance of family relationships for the inner emotional life of the individual. In the years following 1945 it was increasingly recognised that many deprived, maladjusted or delinquent children, criminals, old people and mental patients could not usefully be treated in isolation from their families. In recent years, however, there has been a growing appreciation of the relevance within the family of sociological concepts of role, and a new awareness of the family as a system of interlocking and interacting relationships. Consequently social workers have begun to explore the possibility of applying to their casework with families some of the established methods of working with small groups. The collected articles in *Social Work with Families* (Younghusband, 1965) illustrate this development and show its important implications, both for diagnosis and treatment.

Many children's departments have now accepted that it is part of their function to offer long-term support in the community to socially handicapped families. This has led to obvious difficulties in defining the boundaries of their work and it has also raised problems connected with internal organisation. The wider the range of functions carried out by an individual worker the more difficult is the problem of determining priorities. A child care officer faced with simultaneous demands from an adolescent foster child at crisis point, a baby needing reception into care, and a mother with insufficient cash for the family's weekend food will find the problem of conflicting needs for her time difficult to resolve. Moreover, many child care officers do not feel they have the qualities necessary to bear the depressing confusion and chaos common to many families with multiple problems and at the same time to face the long-term, intensive casework involved.

Some authorities have tried to solve these problems relating to priorities and to individual aptitude by the appointment of separate family caseworkers. This solution has many advantages, including the opportunities for specialist attention to be directed to this group of clients and for new techniques of work with them to be evolved. There can, however, be no rigid frontier between 'family casework' and 'child care'. Children are received into care from and return to the families receiving support from the family caseworkers: a period in care is often both preceded and followed by work with the natural family. Families with multiple problems do not constitute a separate category with sharply defined boundary lines. All child care officers are inevitably concerned with family casework and any specialisation is a matter of emphasis rather than differentiation of function.

Casework with families is too large a subject to be considered in detail in this book; it is in any case the subject of another volume in this series. Mention must however be made of one further aspect of family casework in the context of a children's department. Social casework designed to support and maintain in the community socially handicapped, multi-problem families was initiated by voluntary agencies, notably the Family Service Units. Child care workers are inevitably using their accumulated experience and adopting some of their techniques. There is, however, an important difference. Children's departments have, as we saw earlier in this chapter, statutory protective functions in relation to children in their own homes. A relatively small deterioration in the standards of many of the families receiving long-term casework help will necessitate the exercise of these functions. Some people take the view that the formation of a helpful relationship between the worker and the parent is inhibited by the existence of these legal powers and that the family's caseworker should not be called upon to use them. The possibility that she may do so will, it is argued, reinforce the feelings of hostility to authority which socially handicapped families normally experience. Moreover, a child-centred approach will thereby be introduced into the casework and this will deny the need of the parents to be considered, not only in relation to their children but as people claiming help and attention in their own right. This view implies the introduction of another social worker to the household in the authoritative role if legal action in connection with the children seems necessary, and suggests that such an arrangement would allow the relationship between the family and their caseworker to continue undisturbed.

The proposition described above is superficially attractive but basically unsound because it is not in accordance with the realities of the situation. A caseworker in a statutory setting cannot deny the authority of her agency by avoiding the exercise of this herself. The client will see her not only as an individual but also as a representative of her agency and of the community.

Parents in multi-problem families, perhaps because of their early childhood experiences, often have difficulty in realising that control and concern can be embodied in one person. They tend to distinguish punishing authority figures on the one hand and benign permissive people on the other. In their relationhip with the caseworker, however, they may experience a combination of control and concern which will in itself be corrective and therapeutic.

If this exercise of control involves the caseworker in taking action to remove the children, she will admittedly have no easy task. It will be necessary for her to work through much hostility on the part of the parents and fearfulness and mistrust from the rest of the family. She will have experienced pressures from sections of the community to 'rescue' the children from their 'bad' home, and she will feel guilty that her efforts to keep the family together have not met with success. It is important, however, that she continues to show a concern for and acceptance of the parents as people, together with a belief in the positive aspects of their relationship with the children. Her previous work with the family will have demonstrated her concern that they continue as a unit, and will help her to nurture continuing contact and communication between parents and children. It will also enable them to work with her towards their re-establishment as a group in the community.

# 3

# Reception into care

*Background*

A child may come into the care of the children's committee of a county or a county borough in two main ways; through an application under section 1 of the Children Act 1948 by his parents or by the person who is for the time being looking after him, or following an order made by a juvenile court committing him to the care of the local authority, under the Children and Young Persons Act 1933. A very small proportion (less than 1%) find their way into care by four other routes: these are briefly described later in the chapter.

In the year ending 31st March 1966, 54,000 children came into the care of local authorities in England and Wales, and 52,000 were discharged from care. By comparison, the number of children in care on any one day was only 69,000. This high turnover of children passing in and out of care compared with numbers in care at a point in time reflects the considerable proportion whose period in care is brief. Nearly all these short-term children are received into care under the Children Act 1948: indeed almost exactly half of the total of 54,000 were admitted because of a parent's short-term illness or confinement.

23

On the other hand, the relatively small numbers of children coming into care through the courts remain in care for longer periods: thus, although less than one in ten of the children passing into care during the year are the subjects of juvenile court orders, on any given day one in every three children in care has been committed by a juvenile court.

As these figures show, a small proportion of the children who come into care remain the responsibility of the children's department for a long period, perhaps the whole of their childhood; the rest will stay for only a few weeks or a few months during a temporary family crisis. It is because the population of children in care is constantly changing that the processes of receiving children into care and arranging for their discharge represent a large part of the work of a child care officer.

*Legal provisions*

*The Children Act 1948, Section 1.* The first part of the first section of this Act provides

> where it appears to a local authority with respect to a child in their area appearing to them to be under the age of seventeen—
>
> (a) that he has neither parent nor guardian or has been and remains abandoned by his parents or guardian or is lost; or
>
> (b) that his parents or guardian are, for the time being or permanently, prevented by reason of mental or bodily disease or infirmity or other incapacity or any other circumstances from providing for his proper accommodation, maintenance and upbringing; and

(c) in either case, that the intervention of the local authority under this section is necessary in the interests of the welfare of the child,

it shall be the duty of the local authority to receive the child into their care under this section.

Three points about this section should be noted. Firstly, children may only be received into care if they appear to be under the age of seventeen. The word 'appear' implies that it is not necessary for a child care officer to go to the lengths of inspecting a birth certificate before accepting the child. Secondly, the child must be within the area of the local authority at the time of reception into care. A child who is normally resident in a county in the South of England and who goes during his mother's illness to stay with relatives in a northern city must be received into care in the North if the relatives cannot keep him and he cannot return home. There is, however, provision in the Act for his home county to take over responsibility for his care at a later date if this seems desirable. Thirdly, all children coming into care under this section are 'received' into care. Departments have no power under the Children Act to go out and 'take' children from their parents, even though this may seem to be in the interests of the child.

Section 1 of the Children Act 1948, therefore, makes provision for children in a wide variety of circumstances: the child whose mother has died, has deserted the family, is physically incapacitated or is a patient in a mental hospital; the child whose mother is unmarried and is unable to provide a home; the children whose parents have been evicted from their house and cannot find even temporary accommodation; those with mothers in hospital for the birth of another baby. Children may come into care under this section at a few days old or shortly before their seventeenth birthday; they may be in care for only two days during a temporary family crisis or they may remain in care for up to eighteen years.

It has been possible for local authorities to interpret the wording of this section in different ways according to their policy and the needs of their areas. It is, therefore, important for the child care officer to know the policy and attitude of her department. Some departments treat reception into care as a process which must be avoided if any other alternative is possible. Others may encourage parents to apply rather than to place their children in unsatisfactory private foster homes. Some authorities insist on fathers giving up work to care for young children during their wife's confinement even if the family is in debt and further employment prospects are uncertain: others agree to receive children for short periods during times of crisis in the hope that long-lasting family break-up may be averted. Some children's officers consider the words 'or any other circumstances' cover small children who are deeply rejected by their parents and whose reception into care may prevent long-term emotional damage and maladjustment. Others will not receive a child who has a home and a mother who is providing adequate physical care. The combination of divergent policies with variations in local circumstances is reflected in the different proportions per thousand of the population under eighteen years who are in care of local authorities: for example, in Bootle the figure is 2·6, compared with 10·7 in Bournemouth. It is 9·4 in Oxfordshire and only 2·7 in Devon (H.M.S.O. 1966a). Possible reasons for these differences are explored in Packman (1968).

*The Children and Young Persons Act 1933.* This Act, as amended by sections of the Children and Young Persons Act 1963, provides that juvenile court magistrates may commit to the care of a 'fit person' a child or young person of ten years or over who has been found guilty of an offence which would be punishable in an adult by imprisonment. Courts may also make 'fit person' orders in respect of children who have been found to be in need of care, protection or control. The definition of 'care, protection or control' cannot be given here in full, but it will be found in section 2 of the 1963 Children and Young Persons Act. It includes children who have been neglected, illtreated, assaulted or whose parents have been convicted of offences against other youngsters, and children who have been 'falling into bad associations', are exposed to moral danger or are beyond the control of their parent or guardian.

The 'fit person' may be a relative or friend who is willing to undertake the care of the child but in nearly all cases it is the local authority acting through its children's committee. In each year about one quarter of the children placed in the care of local authorities by juvenile courts have committed offences and about three-quarters are in need of care, protection or control. A 'fit person' order remains in force until its subject has attained the age of eighteen years if the court has not in the meantime revoked the order.

Section 5 of the 1948 Children Act requires local authorities to act as 'fit person' if the court wishes them to do so, unless there is a concurrent probation or supervision order. Children who come into care through the juvenile court are therefore sometimes referred to as section 5 cases. There is, however, considerable divergence of practice in

27

the use of 'fit person' orders by juvenile courts. This order is, of course, only one of many open to the magistrates when they are considering the future of the child before them: alternatives may be an approved school, a probation hostel, a probation or supervision order. If, however, the magistrates decide to make a 'fit person' order they must consider any representations the local authority may wish to make, unless to do so would cause unnecessary delay. Some children's officers are reluctant to accept the fifteen or sixteen year-old who has committed an offence or who is in moral danger and may inform the court that they have no suitable accommodation available for young people in these circumstances. Other children's departments have experimented successfully with special hostel provision and foster homes for the delinquent or near delinquent teenager and have encouraged courts to commit these youngsters to their care rather than to an approved school. Here again the child care officer representing the department in the juvenile court needs to be aware of committee policy and the kind of provision available.

A very small proportion of children come into care of local authority children's committees under the following four provisions.

*The Matrimonial Causes Act 1965* and *The Matrimonial Proceedings (Magistrates' Courts) Act 1960.* These two Acts empower judges dealing with applications for divorce, and magistrates hearing matrimonial complaints to provide for any child of the family to be committed to the care of the local authority. Orders made by courts under these Acts continue in force until the child has attained the age of eighteen years, unless they are in the meantime revoked.

*The Children Act 1948, Section 6(4)*. This section enables local authorities, at the request of the managers of an approved school, to receive into care a child who is released by and under the supervision of the managers if the child has no home of his own or if the managers consider that his home is unsatisfactory. The provision is very little used but it can be of help to certain children from time to time. Since the child becomes the joint responsibility of the managers and of the children's committee, good communication and agreement over plans for him are essential.

*The Children Act 1948, Section 3(4)*. Local authorities may, in some circumstances, assume the rights of parents over children in their care under section 1 of the Act. The procedure will be discussed in the next chapter. This section enables them to receive the children back into their care after discharge if such action appears to be in the interests of the welfare of the child.

*The need for short-term reception into care*

Reference has already been made to the high proportion of children who come into care for short periods during the illness or confinement of their parent. Our increasing knowledge about the effects of separation experiences on small children suggests that the decision to remove them from home for even a short time needs considerable thought. However, two factors handicap the child care officer in her attempts to prevent unnecessary admissions in these cases. The first is the emergency nature of much short stay work. In many instances the department has only two or three days or even hours notice of the child's need for care. Many of these emergencies are unnecessary

29

since investigation often shows that the parents themselves and often a health visitor, teacher or doctor have been aware of the impending crisis for some time. Conscious efforts to persuade the general public and social and medical agencies to approach the department at an early stage can prevent the need for some, though of course not all, emergency work. The second factor is the shortage in many areas of domiciliary services such as home helps, reliable daily minders and day nurseries which could avert the need for many children to come into short-term care. The growing practice of retaining women in hospital for only two or three days following confinement may, in due course, reduce the need to receive their children into care.

The question, however, arises why it is necessary for parents to seek the help of the local authority during these family crises. The 'normal' family is perhaps expected to have relatives or friends who are available in times of difficulty. It would be valuable if research could ascertain the kind of family from which children are received into short-term care. It may be that many have parents whose social mobility has weakened the ties of the wider family and made less available the support traditionally given by them on these occasions. Possibly in some areas substitute care provided by the children's committee is readily offered as a social service and, for this reason, chosen by parents who could make alternative arrangements. The experience of many child care workers would, however, seem to indicate that a high proportion of families needing help at such times have more than the usual quota of problems and inadequacies. In some cases the parents were themselves brought up in substitute care or are at odds with their own relatives; while many are experiencing a degree of social isolation which precludes neighbourly assistance. An application for care of the two and three-year-olds during the third confinement may prove to be the children's department's first introduction to a family which will need social work help for years to come. Application for repeated reception into care may indeed be one of the symptoms of the socially handicapped family comparable with rent arrears, poor school attendance, delinquency or child neglect.

### The parent and the child care officer

The large annual turnover of children in the care of local authorities means that receiving children into care and accepting those who have been committed by the courts, is part of the child care officer's normal routine; the bread and butter work of any children's department. To the child and the parent involved, however, this is always a dramatic experience, a time of confusion and uncertainty when strong and complicated emotions are aroused. The child care officer has to be freshly aware of these feelings in her clients while she is exploring with them the need for reception into care. She must, for instance, bear in mind that at moments of crisis an element of panic often makes it difficult for people to think constructively about their problems. Thus, a mother who has strongly denied any possibility of help from relatives or friends during her hospital admission may well be able to see her own answer to the problem once her anxiety about herself and the children is recognised and she has been assured of help if this becomes necessary. If, on the other hand, an application for care is refused with the situation still unresolved, a 'battle' can develop between the parent and the child care officer in which the needs of the child are overlooked while the parent triumphantly demonstrates as impossible each suggestion made for dealing with the crisis.

Any application for care must in fact be treated as an exploration with the parents of the possible future plans for their child in the light of the resources of the department and the total family position. The feelings and attitudes of parents and child are no less important than the more easily ascertainable facts. Sometimes an application for care may be seen as an appeal for help in a situation that has become unbearable. The applicant seems to be saying 'I can't cope with the housework, with our debts, with my husband, with my depressed unhappy feelings; I am a bad mother, you can do better for the children than I can. Take them and let me be a little girl again.' Both the longing to be dependent and a fear of dependency together with feelings of having somehow failed to act as 'good parents', 'reliable providers' lie buried beneath many applications for children to be received into care. These feelings may be expressed in terms of hostility to the social worker, depressed hopelessness, or apparent unconcern. Moreover, because many of the families asking for this kind of help with their children have experienced a certain amount of social disapproval perhaps from the rent collector, the education welfare officer, officials of the Ministries of Labour and Social Security, they tend to be both resentful and fearful of 'the authorities'.

The child care officer, both as a representative of authority and as one who takes children away and returns them, is an immensely powerful person to the parents in this situation; they may indeed have unexpressed fears that she will prove a modern Pied Piper and that the children will never return home again.

The investigation of an application for care, therefore,

lays the foundation of the department's future relationship with the parents. It is at this stage that they can be helped to see what value the child care officer places on them, what will be expected of them as parents if the child comes into care, and what the department can offer to their child. If an atmosphere is created in which their anxieties and also their desire to act as good parents are recognised, their fears that their son or daughter may be swept up by a large and powerful machine may be dispelled. They can be encouraged to look realistically at the alternatives for their child in care or out of care and a feeling of shared concern for the child will be established.

The parent whose child has just been committed to care by a juvenile court does of course feel particularly anxious and unworthy. The very fact of the committal has by implication labelled him an 'unfit' person. Most parents in these circumstances have only a confused idea of the significance of the court proceedings and this, coupled with the lack of space in many courts, makes the occasion unpropitious for a child care officer to make a first contact. As a minimum, however, it is necessary to explain clearly what has happened and to talk about immediate plans for the child. It is also important to show both the parent and the child that in spite of all that has taken place in the courtroom, their relationship with each other will be valued and recognised by the department.

*Recording*

One of the important functions of a child care officer at this stage, before the child comes into care, is to record as full a picture as possible of the child's development and relationships. The extent to which this is possible depends upon the time available and the place. An emergency reception into care from a police station at midnight does not provide the conditions for a long relaxed talk about a toddler's birth history and early feeding difficulties. If the child has come into care in an emergency these details need to be obtained as soon as possible afterwards. But the children's department needs a full and accurate case history of every child coming into their care. This applies both to long and short-term children, since what appears likely to be a brief period in care often becomes prolonged. Parents, in spite of everyone's efforts, may drop out of a child's life and then precious information is lost. For children living with their own parents there is a collective family memory. A wealth of incident surrounds the day they first went on to 'solids', their first few steps, the time they had their tonsils out. But for children in care this memory has to be artificially created in the children's department's records. These serve another function too. The small child cannot easily keep in touch with all the other people in his life who are important to him—'his sisters, and his cousins and his aunts'. Full record needs to be made of these people, of their relationship to him and of where they can be found. Children who come into care too often lose not only their parents and their parents' memories about their early life, but also the whole range of relatives, friends, teachers, acquaintances who have been the framework of their existence. Sometimes years after a child has come into care someone will tell a child care officer 'if only I'd known at the time I'd have given him a home—or anyway, kept in touch with him'. Many of the lost, isolated children in children's homes with no one in the community who writes to or visits them are in this situation because the living network of relationships which surrounded them at the time they first came into care was not captured on paper and placed in the files for later use. Another important aspect of record keeping at this important pre-reception stage is the noting of details about a child's way of living which will help people who are going to look after him. This is obviously most important for the baby and very young child whose houseparent or foster parent needs to know about routines of feeding, bathing, going to bed. It is also important for older children, because they can thereby have some assurance that thought has been given to their needs and preferences and that their continuing identity as individuals remains safe through changes in external circumstances.

## The child and the child care officer

Mention has already been made of the feelings and anxieties of parents at this time of reception into care, but so far little has been said about the child himself. The way in which he sees reception into care and the impact it has on him will, of course, depend to a great extent on the age and stage he has reached. It is, however, certain that the child's picture of the situation at any age is unrecognisably different from the description of events in departmental case records. The child care officer may see the need for care as arising from a mother's long-planned admission to hospital. The toddler's picture may have a magical flavour. The butterfly in the *Just So Stories* stamped and the palace disappeared. So the child may believe reception into care, the disappearance of his familiar world, to be the direct result of his anger at some small frustration. The child care officer may record another reception in terms of accumulated rent arrears, eviction

35

and the lack of accommodation for all the children concerned in a hostel for homeless families. The twelve-year-old involved may feel he has a partial responsibility for the break-up of the home and may interpret his admission to care as punishment or rejection by his parents.

Similarly, the child care officer may know the 'Laurels' Children's Home is twenty miles away on quite a good bus route: the child may be sure that he is going to the other end of the world and that his father will never find him. The child care officer may know that his mother will be out of hospital in a fortnight's time and back at home again: to the three-year-old a fortnight is not a measurable span of time. So the child care officer may help the child by trying to see a little of his picture and by trying to make clear some of the confusions in it. Small children and dull children may need to have the situation explained over and over again. All children will need factual information presented in a way they can understand. They will also need to show that they are unhappy about what is happening to them. The child care officer is perhaps the only one who can help them by allowing them for a time to be sad, resentful, angry. The parents will find this difficult because of their own feelings about the separation; neighbours and friends will exhort the child to be good, to 'have a lovely holiday', to cheer up; the people to whom the child is going will need to feel that they are being successful in the care they offer. The child care officer can make a space and a time for the child to show some of his real feelings about the situation and she can demonstrate that these are acceptable.

*Pressures on the child care officer*

For the child care officer the process of investigating an

application for care brings pressures from many different sources. She is aware that the decision to separate a child from his home has serious implications, yet other agencies may be pressing her to receive into care before she has been able to make a proper assessment of the situation. She may occasionally find herself in conflict with the policy of her department, considering reception to be in the best interests of the child and yet prevented from arranging this. She may be aware that the only available foster homes or children's homes will fall far short of the child's needs, yet see no alternative to his removal from home; vacancies indeed may be so scarce that it is a matter of searching for any unoccupied bed. There will also be more subtle strains. Parental pressure for a child to be received may rouse conflicting feelings in the child care officer. She will be reluctant to appear an ungiving person; part of her will want to step in and arrange care for the child, to 'solve' the problem, to 'straighten things out'. She may, however, also feel half fearful of the power she has to effect change in external circumstances, hesitant to be the agent through whom the close tie between parent and child is broken.

The temptation is to seek relief from these pressures in constant activity; nevertheless in giving time to understanding the needs of the child and his family at the point of reception into care the child care officer is carrying out one of her most important functions.

# 4

# The child in care and his family

## Working with parents

In the last chapter it was suggested that the foundations of work with children in care and with their parents are laid during the time the child is still in his own home. At this stage the child care officer may help both parent and child to look at the future in the light of the kind of care the department will be able to offer. Where a parent is applying for his child to be received into care, discussion will enable the parent to decide whether this is the best alternative for his child. When it seems possible or probable that the magistrates may make a 'fit person' order, any discussion that can take place about the child's immediate future and what would happen in the event of an order being made will reduce some of the anxieties of the situation.

The extent of the period for which plans must be made can, of course, vary considerably. An infant who is received at the age of ten days old may be in care for all but eighteen years and then continue to receive financial assistance towards the expenses of his maintenance, education or training (Children Act 1948, section 20 as amended by Children and Young Persons Act 1963). Alternatively, he may remain in care for no longer than a week. The amount of time the child will spend in care may be relatively clear and defined at the outset or it may be indefinite: discharge may depend on a mother coming out of hospital following the birth of a baby, or on the remote possibility of evicted parents while the resolution is still effective; indeed the duration of the period for which care is required is of course a necessary element in discussions with parents about a child's future.

How far parents are able to share in making realistic plans for their child will bear some relation to their intelligence and emotional maturity: it will depend on their capacity for looking ahead; on their ability to see the child as an individual with needs differentiated from their own; on the extent to which they have been able to come to terms with the separation and with the role of the local authority. Whatever stage of development they have reached, however, it is essential that they are involved to the limit of their capacities in any consideration of the future; this both follows from and demonstrates a recognition of the important and unique place they hold in a child's life.

These considerations apply whatever the route by which a child has come into care, whether or not the parents have been considered 'good' or 'bad', 'fit' or 'unfit'. They are even to some extent independent of the legal position. But a proper understanding of the duties and powers of the local authority in relation to parents is nevertheless essential in any process of considering the future of children in care.

## Legal position of parents under the Children Act 1948

Section 1(3) of the Children Act states: 'Nothing in this

39

section shall authorise a local authority to keep a child in their care under this section if any parent or guardian desires to take over the care of the child.' The section goes on to make it clear that the local authority must, where it appears to them consistent with the welfare of the child, endeavour to secure that the parent takes over his care. If, therefore, the parents of a child in care under section 1 of the Children Act 1948 do not agree with the way in which the authority is providing for him, they may resume care themselves. While he remains in care, however, they have no right to determine where he shall reside or by whom he shall be looked after. The local authority, for their part, have no right to make decisions which are legally those of a parent: they cannot give consent to the child having an operation, they cannot change his religion, they cannot agree to his marriage. Most children's departments at the stage of reception into care take the precaution of asking parents to sign an agreement authorising the local authority to consent to emergency medical and dental treatment on their behalf.

For the majority of children coming into care under the Children Act, the legal position between local authority and parent remains at this level of voluntary agreement. It is, however, possible in certain defined circumstances for the local authority to resolve to take over all the rights and powers of the parent or guardian. Section 2 of the 1948 Children Act as amended and extended by section 48 of the Children and Young Persons Act 1963, defines the grounds on which such a resolution may be taken. These are:

(a) that his parents are dead and that he has no guardian: or

(b) that a parent or guardian of his (hereinafter referred to as the person on whose account the resolution was passed) has abandoned him, or suffers from some permanent disability rendering the said person incapable of caring for the child, or is of such habits or mode of life as to be unfit to have the care of the child, or suffers from a mental disorder (within the meaning of the Mental Health Act 1959 or the Mental Health (Scotland) Act 1960), which renders him unfit to have the care of the child; or has so persistently failed without reasonable cause to discharge the obligations of a parent or guardian as to be unfit to have the care of the child.

Parents whose wherabouts have remained unknown to the local authority having care of their children for twelve months or more are considered to have abandoned their children, and, under another section of the 1948 Act, a duty is placed on parents of children in care under sixteen years of age to keep the local authority informed of their address.

Once a local authority has passed a resolution under section 2 of the Children Act 1948 the parent or parents must be formally notified and they have a right to object to the resolution. If they do this then the resolution lapses unless the authority complains to a juvenile court and the court upholds the local authority's action. If the parents do not object, or if the court upholds the resolution, then the local authority retains the rights and powers of parents until the child is eighteen years old or until the resolution is rescinded by the authority themselves or by a juvenile court. The powers of a parent to change a child's religion or to consent to his adoption are specifically excluded from the authority's rights under this section, but apart from this they are legally in the position of the parents. They may, if they wish, allow the child to go to live with his own parents while the resolution is still effective; indeed this is frequently arranged if the circumstances at home have improved and there is a possibility that the resolution may be rescinded if the child settles satisfactorily.

In 1963 about one-fifth of children in care under section I of the Children Act 1948 were subjects of resolutions under section 2 of the Act. The extent to which these resolutions are taken varies considerably from one authority to another. Some children's committees make considerable use of them and consider that the legal grounds on which they may be passed should be extended. Broadly, however, with the increasing emphasis on working with parents to achieve a mutually agreed plan, child care thinking would support the view that parental rights should only be taken where this is absolutely necessary to protect the interests of the child.

As we have seen, the other main route by which children come into care is through the juvenile court.

*Legal position of parents in 'fit person' cases*

Section 75(4) of the Children and Young Persons Act 1933 provides that the person to whose care a child or young person is committed on a 'fit person' order 'shall, while the order is in force, have the same rights and powers . . . as if he were his parent, and the person so committed shall continue in his care notwithstanding any claim by a parent or any other person'. This places local authorities acting as 'fit person' in substantially the same position vis-à-vis parents as with section 2 resolutions. The 'fit person' order remains in force until the child is eighteen years old or until it is revoked by a juvenile court. Again, the authority may allow the child to live with his own parents while the order is running and again they are not empowered either to change the child's religion or to consent to his adoption.

## Parental contributions to child's maintenance

This is an important aspect of a local authority's relationship with the parents of children in care. Whether the child has come into care under section 1 of the Children Act, or under the Children and Young Persons Act 1933, the father and the mother too, if she has a separate income, are liable to contribute to his maintenance until he attains the age of sixteen years. After this age the child himself can be asked to make contributions for his own keep if he is in 'remunerative full-time work'. Step-parents have no liability to maintain. The father and mother are assessed by the local authority to contribute an amount determined by their means. If they fall into arrears the authority may apply to a magistrates court for a contribution order. The magistrates will then decide the amount payable and may provide that it is to be deducted from the parents' wages. It is within the power of the magistrates to commit a parent to prison if payments are not made on a court order.

The assessment and collection of parental contributions is in many authorities almost completely separate from other aspects of the work of a children's department. It is usually the concern of administrative rather than social work staff, and except in certain special cases the emphasis is on overall fairness and similarity of treatment rather than on catering for individual circumstances and needs.

The parent himself will not of course make this distinction between the child care and financial aspects of his relationship with the department. His attitude to the payment of money for his children's keep will often express and reflect his feelings about his children and the local authority's caring for them; he may, for instance, miss several weeks' payments because he feels the housemother has been unwelcoming or critical when he visits. This is an area of potential conflict between the social worker and the administrator. The child care officer may be encouraging a parent to pay off accumulated debts for rent in order to re-establish his home and take his children out of care. At the same time, independently the father may be receiving letters from the office dealing with parental contributions, making it clear that court action will follow if he does not keep up his payments. Effective communications between administrative and fieldwork staff is essential in the interest of the client.

This account of various aspects of the legal relationship between the children's committee and the parents of children in care has shown both the limits and the extent of the local authority's powers. It should be emphasised that the resources of the authority in terms of legal knowledge and experience are enormous: the parent is often an inadequate person whose life experience has made him suspicious and apprehensive of the court and the Town Hall. The possibilities for official 'hoodwinking' of parents are very great and such methods may sometimes appear to be in the interests of the children. They can, however, in the long run only damage these interests. It is important that parents have their legal rights fully explained to them when they are at issue with the authority and that apparently irreconcilable conflicts are decided by a court. However, as stated above, the establishment at the outset of a relationship where parents feel valued by the authority and are brought into discussion of plans for their children will reduce the number of conflicts of this kind.

*The plan*

What factors must be taken into account in making plans with and for a child in care? To begin with, the assessment is not only of the child but also of his situation; it is an assessment of the child within the network of his past and present relationships. Secondly, it is an assessment not only of the present but also of the future; an attempt to estimate how long the child will remain in care and how the people in his life are going to act and feel in relation to him and to each other. Thirdly, it is an assessment of the resources of the organisation which is caring for him; an examination of the various possibilities in terms of the child's present and future needs.

The same basic considerations apply whether a child is received into care for an indefinite period or for no longer than ten days. Children who have been committed to care by a juvenile court or those whose stay is likely to be prolonged are usually admitted to a reception centre where these assessments can be made before a long-term placement is arranged, and where psychiatric, medical and psychological help in diagnosis may be available. Most children who come into care do so, however, for short periods and are placed directly in foster homes, nurseries or children's homes. In these cases the child care officer has to try to carry out some of the assessment functions of the reception centre during her visits to the home before the child is received. She must therefore with the help of the parents and from her own observation attempt to form a clear picture of the child's development, physical condition, behaviour, feelings, relationships and interests. This will both facilitate a wise decision about his placing and enable housemother or foster mother to go some way towards indentifying, understanding and meeting his needs.

Whatever the likely duration of a child's stay in care the decision about where to place him is rarely an easy one. This is because the resources of the department are limited and each child has a unique combination of needs. Thus a boy may need to remain near to his own village; to receive continuing visits from an aggressive father; to live in the catchment area of a school for educationally subnormal children; and to be in a home with no other children of the same age and one which will tolerate his occasional petty pilfering. It would be unusually fortunate if the department had a foster home or children's home which could meet all these needs; surprising if this home had a vacancy for the boy we have described. For this is only one of many children in the care of the department whose needs have to be met, and the interests of the adults and children in the group to which he may be admitted also need consideration. A decision about placement for a child involves both a decision about the priorities of the child's own different needs and also a balancing of the conflicting needs of other children and adults in the situation. An 'ideal' solution for all concerned is rarely a possibility : the best solution will have unsatisfactory aspects.

## The child

We have in this chapter considered some of the factors which must be taken into account when a decision is made about the placement of a child: the legal position of parents has been outlined and the importance of involving them to the limits of their capacity has been stressed. But decisions need to be made, not only about children but also *with* children. The extent to which children in care can enter into plans for their own future does of course depend on their age and stage of development, as well as on their circumstances. The four-year-old going to a foster home may be able to share only in the decision about which of his special belongings he takes with him: the adolescent can perhaps be helped to make a realistic choice from available lodgings. For all children, the sense of sharing in even small decisions can make the situation seem safer and more bearable because some of it is within their control. But the exercising of real choice in relation to large areas of his own future is usually too frightening and burdensome to a child and beyond his capacity. Children's own preferences, which they themselves may not at this stage fully understand, are in complex situations only one of the strands which go to make up the skein. In these instances factual information about plans and proposed arrangements will enable the child to make a picture of the future; he will be helped further if he feels that his attitudes to these proposals can have some real effect on what will happen.

Many children in care have no idea of what is going to happen next: their view of time to come is blocked by a blank wall and their anxiety about this may be so great that they cannot bring themselves to ask what lies on the other side. They are therefore believed to be unconcerned about the future. The child care officer herself may not have any clear idea of what can be arranged, and this will be a pressure on her in discussions with the child. However, even her shared uncertainty conveyed with concern will be more bearable for the child than silence and the fear of the completely unknown. The child care officer is, of course, not the only person in the child's life who will discuss the future with him. His parents, and the people who are for the time being filling parental roles, will perhaps also help him to look ahead. The child care officer has, however, a special contribution because she stands outside the immediate circumstances of his living and for this reason she may enable him to see the picture as a whole.

In the next two chapters we shall discuss the importance to the child who is established in foster or residential care of his relationship with the field worker. However, when movement and change are proposed or recently accomplished, effective communication between child and social caseworker is vital. A good illustration of the way in which a car journey may be used to establish this kind of communication will be found in *The Understanding Caseworker* (Stevenson, 1963). It is during these periods of uncertainty that a child will most clearly demonstrate both his need of and dependence on a relationship with the child care officer: for a relatively short time she will perhaps seem the most important person in his life. She may indeed, as Clare Winnicott (1964) suggests, have to stand in as the good, giving person for him. If her work is to be successful, however, she will enable the child to make or re-establish other relationships with foster parents, residential workers or his own parents. From these relationships the child will be able to enjoy continuous and direct experiences which, because of the nature of her role, the child care officer cannot provide for him. It is sometimes difficult for a child care officer to relinquish her position at the centre of the child's world because this can give her very real satisfactions. Unless she is able to do this, she is failing her child because he will continue to need her in an important but different way. This will be considered further in Chapters 5 and 6.

# 5

# Foster care

*The development of foster care*

The Children Act 1948 provides that local authorities shall maintain a child in a children's home only when it is 'not practicable or desirable for the time being to make arrangements for boarding out'. Children's departments, therefore, have a duty to consider the possibility of fostering for each child in their care. This statutory requirement does not, however, indicate that boarding out is the 'ideal' method of care for each and every child. The Curtis Report drew attention to the dangerous consequences of this way of thinking, and emphasised the importance of having regard to the qualities of individual foster homes and the needs of the particular child. The proposition that foster care is 'better' than residential care is as meaningless as is the contrary.

The essence of fostering for children in care, as defined by the Boarding Out of Children Regulations 1955, is that the child lives with foster parents in their dwelling as a member of their family. Within these limits, however, the nature of foster care has undergone important changes during the years that children's departments have been in existence. If all care outside the child's own family is seen as a continuum, from adoption at one extreme, through children's homes to the approved school at the other, then the function of foster care has moved away from that of near adoption and closer to that of residential care. When children tended to come into the care of local authorities at an early age, to lose touch with their parents and to go out of care at eighteen years old, their needs were for a complete substitute home, a quasi-adoptive situation. The development of family casework, the increasing emphasis on the child in care as a part of his natural family and the resources of staff and time devoted to re-uniting him with his parents as soon as possible have very greatly reduced the proportions of these long-term, near adoptive, fostering situations and have altered the character of foster care.

Natural parents are increasingly encouraged to visit foster homes and the majority of foster parents are now caring for children for short or indeterminate periods: not so many are now regarded as complete parent substitutes and few are able to look confidently ahead to the young child achieving adult status in their home.

Moreover, the greater attention now paid to avoiding wherever possible the need for reception into care, together with the increased number of children committed by juvenile courts, seem in many areas to have reduced the number of relatively stable, 'easy' children available for boarding out. These factors, the limitation on the duration of the fostering period, the greater participation of natural parents and the more serious difficulties presented by foster children, have changed the satisfactions foster parents can now expect to receive and have important indications for their recruitment.

The nature of foster care, then, is influenced by general

child care policies through the effect these have on the needs of children in care, and there is considerable variation between local authorities both in policy and in the way their service has developed. The extent to which foster care is used is also affected by social and economic conditions. Areas which have a tradition of married women working outside the home or where housing is particularly overcrowded will obviously not be favourable to the recruitment of foster homes. This variation between authorities in the use of foster care may be illustrated by official statistics (*Children in Care in England and Wales*, H.M.S.O., Cmnd. 3204, 1966). At 31st March 1966, 51% of all children in care of local authorities in England and Wales were boarded out. The figure for the London Boroughs, however, was only 33%. The proportions ranged from 18% in one authority in central London, to 95% in a rural Welsh County.

These figures do not, of course, indicate that the proportions of children 'suitable for foster care' or the numbers of people who are 'acceptable as foster parents' show a variation of this magnitude between authorities. It is doubtful whether the concept of 'suitability for boarding out' has any value. A child can be boarded out if a foster home is available which suits his needs. Similarly, a foster home is acceptable if it can meet the needs of the child for whom it is intended. The needs referred to may include contact and communication with difficult parents. Some children are extremely hard to foster because they require skilled care, a great deal of attention and physical space. Few foster parents are able to meet these demands and the children are therefore normally accommodated in children's homes. However, some progress has been made over the years in boarding out physically, mentally and emotionally handicapped children, and there is no reason to suppose that we have exhausted the pool of homes in the community able to care for children with exceptional needs. It seems likely that the development of fostering in recent years has been limited both by lack of clarity about the role of the foster parent, and by increasing pressures on child care officers who have had insufficient time to devote to the recruitment and investigation of foster homes.

*The selection of foster parents*

This is without doubt one of the most difficult tasks a child care officer performs. In undertaking a foster home placement, she is creating a network of relationships which can be broken only at the risk of damage to the child and unhappiness to all involved. Yet there are few objective criteria to guide her. In this country research has in the main been confined to relatively small scale studies of foster care in individual local authorities. Two of these projects are, however, of particular importance. Trasler (1960) analysed characteristics of foster homes and foster children in a sample of children in the care of one local authority who were removed from foster homes over a three-year period. Parker (1966) has suggested a prediction table of success and failure in fostering on the basis of research into long-term foster home placements in an English county. He emphasises that the table needs validation with a larger sample of children in areas with different policies and conditions, but his study clearly shows the value of developing predictive techniques as an important tool of the social caseworker in this difficult field. 'Predictive studies can present the combined experience of many workers with many cases in a condensed and tested form,

(Parker *op. cit.*). It is not intended that they shall replace the judgment of the caseworker in a particular case by a mechanised, statistical measure. One or two of Parker's findings may be mentioned here:

(i) The likelihood of a successful placement being made decreased as the age of the child to be boarded out increased. This result is compatible with the conclusions of Trasler.

(ii) The highest rate of failure was found in those placements of children who had spent three years or more in institutions.

(iii) There was a significant continuous decline in the rate of successful fostering with increasing age at separation from mother.

(iv) The presence in the foster home of a son or daughter of the foster parents whose age was within five years of that of the foster child was a prejudicial factor, as was the existence of any natural child of the foster mother under five years of age.

(v) Foster mothers over forty years of age appeared to be most successful, and those under thirty markedly least successful. This also is compatible with the results of other studies.

There are general considerations which will govern the approach of the caseworker to the couple offering themselves as foster parents. She will probably find that her attempts to discover the 'motives' behind the application prove fruitless and misleading. People find it difficult to talk about their reasons for offering a home to a child, and as is well known these are rarely clearly defined or what they superficially appear. It is perhaps more helpful to seek to discover what satisfactions the foster parents hope to gain, what needs in their life they are trying to meet in this situation; to determine whether these expectations are realistic and their needs compatible with those of children for whom the agency is seeking a home. That foster parents, like houseparents and child care officers, have needs which they may legitimately satisfy through children in care is now generally accepted: the idea of a foster mother caring for children out of detached compassion is both unrealistic and unsatisfactory.

It follows that there are some needs which children in care are unlikely to be able to meet. The need to 'mend' a failing matrimonial relationship; the need to 'cure' mental ill-health or to provide companionship for a spoilt only child, are perhaps obvious examples. There are other less easily recognised needs which may prove dangerous if satisfaction is sought for them through a foster child: the need to possess and control; the need of affectionless persons to be reassured of their ability to give and receive affection; the need of those who feel themselves to be unworthy, to gain social approval through the performance of worthy tasks; the need to deal with neurotic feelings of guilt. A desire to experience vicariously unfulfilled ambitions of their own is perhaps common to most parents, but in both natural and foster parents it can be so overwhelming as to deny completely the individuality of the child.

What kind of people are children's departments hoping to recruit as foster parents? Certainly as Clare Winnicott (1964) has pointed out 'we are not looking for perfect parents because they only exist in theory and in fantasy'. Children's departments need foster parents who are already managing to find some satisfactions in their lives and who are dealing reasonably successfully with their problems. These people will probably have certain common charac-

55

teristics: a continuing need 'to parent' which is not being fulfilled; an ability to accept a foster child and his existing network of relationships without denying that he has a past and probably a future in which they have no part; a potential for deriving satisfaction from caring for a child and helping him through a difficult part of his childhood; sufficient flexibility to enable them to rearrange the pattern of their lives so as to include a child they do not know; some capacity for tolerating stress and uncertainty without exhausting the emotional resources of the family.

Within these broad limits there is room in the child care service for foster parents with many different skills and aptitudes. The woman who enjoys caring for a succession of small babies who are awaiting placement for adoption may differ in important respects from the foster mother who has a special talent for dealing with difficult adolescent girls or the foster parents with the insight and staying power to see a maladjusted boy through a period of several years in care. Parker (*op. cit.*) has pointed out that we do not know in what respects successful long-stay foster parents differ from those who can take relays of children for short periods. Research has much to discover in this area, but it is unlikely to reveal a limited number of stereotypes of 'ideal' foster parents.

In the process of investigating a foster parent application the child care officer establishes a relationship with the applicants which lays the foundations of their expectations of the department. She is seeking to discover with them whether some of their needs can be met by a foster child: she is also estimating whether they will be able to work within the framework of the agency. In the initial interviews the giving and receiving of information will necessarily predominate. The child care officer will help the applicants to clarify for themselves the nature of the work for which they are applying; she will try to give them some understanding of the needs of children for whom homes may be required. At this stage and later many applicants will want to withdraw, acknowledging that their ideas about fostering were unrealistic, and they should be helped to do this without feeling guilty or unworthy. The child care officer will also seek information from the applicants. She must, for instance, in accordance with the Boarding Out Regulations, make a written report covering the following points before any child is boarded out in the home: the sleeping and living accommodation and other domestic conditions at the dwelling; the reputation and religious persuasion of the foster parents and their suitability in age, character, temperament and health to have the charge of the child; whether any member of the foster parents' household is believed to be suffering from any physical or mental illness which might adversely affect the child or to have been convicted of any offence which would render it undesirable that the child should associate with him; and the number, sex and approximate age of the persons in the household. Most authorities ask for the names of responsible people, often including the family doctor, who will act as referees; and they will also check with other departments such as police, education and health whether anything is known about the family which would make it inadvisable to place a child with them.

## Boarding-out allowances

Remuneration was not mentioned as one of the needs which may bring a couple to apply to be considered as

foster parents. During the first ten years or so of the existence of children's departments the question of whether
the allowances paid for boarded out children should include an element of profit was hotly debated. The shadow
of the Victorian baby farmer hung over the discussion and
there were those who considered that a desire to earn
money by fostering was not compatible either with the
provision of good care or with feelings of warmth and
affection for the child. Similarly, in the early days of the
nursing profession it was felt that the good nurse must be
'above' an interest in an adequate living wage. Even now,
perhaps those engaged professionally in social work, particularly in its residential aspects, are expected to feel a
sense of dedication which excludes the wish for proper
financial reward. So far as foster parents are concerned
there has been an increasing appreciation of the fact that
they undertake a difficult and time-consuming task for
which payment is not inappropriate. The child care officer
is concerned less with their interest in the financial aspect
than with their reason for choosing to supplement their
income in this particular way. There are, after all, easier
ways of earning money.

Each local authority and voluntary children's society
decides its own scale of boarding-out allowances. These
can reflect differences in the cost of living between one
part of the country and another, and differences in the
satisfactions and difficulties involved in caring for a particular child. A child with few problems who is expected to
remain in a foster home for an indefinite period and to
provide some of the emotional satisfaction of a natural or
adopted child may rate a lower boarding-out allowance
than the maladjusted adolescent with multiple problems
who is placed for a short period. Special allowances for

short stay or particularly difficult children are quite common, and in many cases an element of 'profit' is included. Most authorities operate a scale which provides additional allowances for holidays, special clothing needs, items such as music lessons, or exceptional expenditure on household replacements.

## The child care officer and the foster parent

Mention has already been made of the importance of assessing how well prospective foster parents will be able to accept a role involving shared responsibility for a child. The nature of the relationship between the child care officer as representative of the agency, and the foster parent, is central to the success or failure of a placement. Yet this relationship is difficult to analyse and in some ways unique. Foster parents are neither clients nor colleagues. They are not clients because they have come to the agency offering to undertake a specified task: they have not given the caseworkers sanction to offer help with their personal problems. They are not colleagues because the child care officer has important supervisory functions in regard to them and they are not professional people employed by the society or department. Yet there are occasions when the relationship may closely resemble that between worker and client on the one hand, or between colleagues on the other. Stresses connected or unconnected with the fostering situation may create or reactivate problems in a foster parent with which she needs help. Referral to another agency may not be practicable, the welfare of the foster child may be affected and the child care officer may find herself in a worker-client relationship. Similarly, the foster parent who has worked closely with an agency over a number of years may have acquired an identification with it and an expertise which gives her a colleague-like relationship with the child care officer.

Clare Winnicott (1964, *op. cit.*) has identified three elements in this relationship of child care officer and foster parent: supervisory, supportive and educational. The supervisory aspect was predominant in the early days of boarding out when the poor economic conditions of most working class families made close attention to the foster child's physical well-being of first importance. Recently perhaps child care workers have tended to underplay their supervisory role and seem at times almost to deny it. The foster parent, however, is aware that she stands in a contractual relationship to the agency, and that the child care officer is responsible for ensuring that the terms of this contract are observed. The Boarding Out of Children Regulations require that in each placement which is expected to last for more than eight weeks the foster parent shall sign an undertaking agreeing, among other things, to allow the agency access to the child at all times, to allow the child to be removed from their home by an authorised person (and following perhaps strangely from the last clause) to care for the child and bring him up as they would a child of their own. They also promise to look after the child's health and to encourage him to practise his religion. By the same Regulations the department or agency is required to visit the child at not less than certain stated intervals which vary according to his age and the length of time he has been in the foster home; to review his welfare, health, conduct and progress within three months of boarding out and then not less often than once every six months; to arrange for regular medical examination and any necessary medical and dental attention and to remove him forthwith if the conditions in which he is boarded out endanger his health, safety or morals.

The supervisory aspect is an important element in the relationship, therefore, and should not be denied. The child care officer must accept that in the eyes of the foster parent she is a person with the power to bring a child and to take him away. So threatening in its implication is this power, in fact, that some foster parents try to pretend it does not exist by seeking to establish a relationship with the child care officer which is in essence social rather than professional. The child care officer will in these instances feel that by invitations to meals, by gifts, by a determination to keep conversation on the level of polite chat, the foster mother is manipulating her into the role of a personal friend. There have for some time past been suggestions that foster parents should be given greater protection from decisions by local authorities or parents to remove children from their care. It would not be easy to devise a method which would protect foster parents in this way and yet safeguard the interests of the child and the natural parent. The course of making application for an adoption order in respect of their foster child is always open to foster parents who, if successful, thereby gain full parental rights.

The foster home breakdown is a different matter; here the foster parents either unilaterally or in co-operation with the child care officer decide that they cannot keep the child in their home. Such breakdowns are distressing to all concerned and are liable to arouse guilty feelings in the child care officer who feels she has exposed the child and foster parent to this experience. It is frequently better to accomplish the removal of a child from a foster home before feelings become exacerbated to breaking point in order that a relationship between child and foster parent may be carried over into the next stage of the child's life.

The child care officer's supportive role with foster parents will involve the acknowledgment of shared responsibility for the child, the giving of information about the resources of the department and the assurance that these will be available if required. It will also involve the acceptance of their negative feelings towards the foster child and his natural parents. Foster parents need to feel that it is safe for them to express their irritation, anger and frustration to the child care officer. This discharge of feeling may in itself do much to relieve tensions but it is also a necessary preliminary to the educational processes described in the next paragraph. Strong feelings in the foster parents which have remained unexpressed will be a barrier to their achievement of understanding. The child care officer may find some difficulty in giving foster parents 'permission' to express critical or angry feelings, particularly if she has herself placed the foster child, is indentified with him in the situation, and is very anxious for the placement to be successful. At times of stress foster parents will also need reassurance that their work is valued. After they have expressed negative feelings they may be helped to recognise the positive elements in their relationship with the child and his family.

The educational aspects of the relationship between child care officer and foster parent follow from the child care officer's supportive role, and involve helping the foster parents to understand both the needs of the foster child and their own feelings about the demands he makes on them. The foster family may sometimes find reassurance in the knowledge that actions which they find worrying and inexplicable are within the range of normal behaviour for a child in this situation.

Some departments have reinforced the supportive and educational role of individual child care officers by arranging foster parent meetings and discussion groups or circulating periodic news letters. These give the support of the consciousness of membership of an organisation and also make it possible for foster parents to learn from shared experience with others in the same situation. Foster parents are perhaps by their nature not enthusiastic 'joiners'; they can feel both isolated and lonely. The extent to which they are often a focus of the envious, critical and hostile feelings of neighbours should not be underestimated.

## Foster parents and natural parents

What are the feelings of the child's own parents towards the person who is, for the time being, caring for his child? Much that will be said in the next chapter about the relationship between residential staff and natural parents is of course relevant to this. There is, however, an important difference: the staff of children's homes, nurseries and approved schools are professionals; in the eyes of the parents they are 'experts'. The foster parent in his own home is in some respects what the natural parent might have been; the adequate, coping, socially approved person who has been given the function of remedying deficiencies in the provision available in the child's own home. Foster parents do not perhaps awaken the anti-authority feelings of parents as readily as do houseparents, but they more easily become the focus of their envy and the target of their criticism. The foster parent for his part is likely to experience feelings of antagonism for the natural parent.

It is not easy to share the affections of a child, and the foster parents know that however good their care, the natural parent occupies a place in the child's emotions which they can never supplant. Moreover, there are all the feelings of the hard-working, conscientious elder brother toward the prodigal son. The respectable, widowed mother with a physical illness can expect compassion from the foster parents, but her children rarely perhaps find their way into care: the happy-go-lucky, improvident, ne'er-do-well father or promiscuous mother who visit the foster home and depart in a haze of sentiment, leaving the foster mother with the hard realities of washing, bathing and putting to bed, may awaken the anger that contains an element of envy. An important function of the child care officer is to help both the natural parent and the foster parent to express and understand their feelings in relation to each other; to interpret and to clarify without appearing to take sides or to defend.

## The child care officer and the foster child

Again, much that will be said in the next chapter about the function of the child care officer with children in residential care applies in the case of foster children. But again there are important differences. The supervisory element in the role of the child care officer in the foster home can make her contact with the child a threat to the foster mother. For this reason it is important for child care officers to make it clear to foster parents, before ever a child is placed with them, that they will need to have a direct relationship with him and that this need does not spring primarily from an anxiety about the treatment he will receive. There are those who believe that once a 'satisfactory' foster placement has been made it is unnecessary and damaging for the child care officer to establish direct communication with the child. This denies the need of children in care for a casework relationship which clarifies and contains their life experience. This point will be developed further in the next chapter. Certainly, the difficulty for the child care officer in making contact with a foster child she has not herself placed and whose foster parents are suspicious and resentful is not easily overcome. Here much careful work with the foster parents is necessary in order to establish their confidence in the child care officer's appreciation of their worth and importance before effective communication with the child can be achieved.

So far in this chapter consideration has been given to those foster children who are in the care of local authorities or voluntary societies. Brief mention must now be made of the children's committee's duty towards children not in care who are living apart from their parents in private homes.

*Children fostered privately under the Children Act 1958*

Part 1 of this Act is concerned with children of compulsory school age and under, whose care and maintenance are undertaken for reward for a period exceeding one month by a person who is not a relative or guardian. Children who are the responsibility of public or local authorities are specifically excluded from these provisions. The local authority is given the duty of arranging for these private foster children to be visited from time to time by officers who must satisfy themselves as to the well-being of the children and give such advice on their care and maintenance as may appear to be needed. A person proposing to receive a foster child in these circumstances is legally obliged to notify the local authority in writing two weeks beforehand, unless the placement is made in an emergency, and the authority is given powers to inspect the premises, and if necessary to prohibit their use. In some instances the authority may impose limits on the number of foster children kept and require the maintenance of certain standards of care. Certain people, including those who have been convicted of offences against children, are disqualified from acting as foster parents unless the local authority specifically agrees to them doing so. Authorities may, if they consider that a child is about to be received or is being kept in a detrimental environment or by a person unfit to have his care, complain to a Justice of the Peace or a juvenile court for an order empowering them to remove the child to a place of safety.

At 31st March 1966, over 10,000 children were being supervised by local authorities under this Act. Little is known about the home backgrounds of these private foster children, whether application was ever made for them to be received into care, or why they are living apart from their parents. It seems probable, however, that in the Home Counties at any rate, a high proportion are the children of immigrants, particularly Africans and West Indians, who are studying or working in this country. These parents often have little knowledge of English cultural and social standards and tend to be undiscriminating in their choice of foster homes; consequently there are grounds for concern about the care received by some of their children. Illegitimate children awaiting adoption placement by voluntary adoption societies are also commonly placed in private foster homes. The element of reward, that is payment in cash or in kind, is central in the definition of foster children under this Act. It sometimes happens that a parent is unable to continue to make payments for his child and application is made to the local authority for the child to be received into care.

## Protected children under the Adoption Act 1958

Protected children, as defined by Part 4 of the Adoption Act, fall into two main categories. Those in respect of whom there is intention to apply for an adoption order are one group who will be considered in Chapter 7. The other group who may never become involved in adoption proceedings consists of those of compulsory school age and under who are placed with people who are not relatives or guardians and someone who is not the parent or guardian takes part in the arrangements. Again, children in the care of public authorities or voluntary children's societies are excluded. The essential element in the definition of a protected child under section 37(a) of the Adoption Act is that a third party, not a parent or guardian, has taken part in arrangements made to place him with an unrelated person. There is no element of reward for his care and maintenance as in the case of private foster children who may be placed directly by their own parents. Under the Adoption Act local authorities have similar powers to inspect premises and prohibit the placing of children as they have in the case of private foster children. They also have similar duties to secure that the children are visited by staff who will satisfy themselves as to their well-being. Whereas in the case of private foster children the onus to report the placement is on the foster parent herself, in the case of protected children the third party making the arrangements is legally required to notify the local authority.

It will be noted that whereas children placed by their parents for reward become foster children, and children placed by a third party become protected children, those children who are placed with strangers by their parents without any payment being made are excluded from both these categories. Children's departments, in fact, have no special powers or duties in respect of this group. A mother may still give her baby to a stranger in a bus queue without any public authority having the right to enquire into the arrangement.

## Children fostered privately and protected children

The legal and administrative differences between children boarded out by local authorities and voluntary societies on the one hand and protected children and private foster children on the other should not obscure the similarity of their needs in what is, from the standpoint of the child, essentially the same position. Private foster children and protected children have the same uncertainties, the same confusions as children in care, and they need the same kind of casework help. It is, however, often difficult for the supervising child care officer to give this because her relationship with the foster mother differs in important respects. So far as these foster parents are concerned, the children's department has decided not to prohibit an arrangement already made for them to receive the child, it has not provided them with a child, together with an invisible badge of official approval as in the case of 'official' foster parents. In most cases the people undertaking to care for the children will not at the outset be aware of the department's interest in the arrangement and the child care officer will appear as an unwelcome inspector: a role which social workers do not find easy. From the child care officer's standpoint her powers are here less clearly defined, her detailed duties less explicit: the two weeks' statutory notice of placement is rarely long enough for her to do more than exclude the most obviously unsuitable homes. The difficulties are therefore greater, the needs similar. Where it is possible to overcome the initial hostility and suspicion of private foster parents and those looking after protected children the child care officer may be able to offer valuable help to the child, the foster parent and the natural parent.

# 6

# Residential care

*Development and present function*

Residential care, no less than foster care, must be seen in the context of total provision for children in need of help. An increase or decrease in the ratio of children boarded out, the development of new techniques in work with families, a change in the policy of juvenile courts, could each affect the size and character of the population in approved schools, children's homes and hostels. Thus, both the amount and type of residential provision is influenced by local need and local policy. As we have already observed in connection with the boarding out statistics, there is considerable variation between authorities. Whereas 39% of all children in care of children's committees in England and Wales are accommodated in children's homes and nurseries (*Children in Care in England and Wales*, Cmnd. 3204), there were at 31st March 1966, no children at all in this form of care in Montgomeryshire and 65% in the London Borough of Haringey. There is a similar variation in the numbers of children maintained by local authorities in approved schools.

It will not be possible, for reasons of space, to give detailed consideration in this book to approved schools and remand homes. Nevertheless, the fact that they constitute an important part of residential child care provision must not be overlooked. All remand homes, and just under a quarter of the approved schools, in this country are provided by children's committees. Local authorities have a liability to contribute to the maintenance of children from their area in approved schools and they share with the probation service a responsibility for after-care.

Although children's departments are closely involved with approved schools and remand homes, these have developed largely in isolation from children's homes, reception centres and hostels. Residential schools for maladjusted children, the responsibility of the education service, form another separate group. Yet these three types of residential establishment have much in common. Some children experience all these forms of treatment during the first seventeen years of their life and it is indeed arguable that the corresponding adjectives 'delinquent', 'maladjusted', 'deprived', are descriptive of administrative and legal categories rather than of fundamental differences in need and behaviour. Moreover, the problems and techniques of caring for children in a group are not substantially different in the three settings; and each has the same broad purpose of helping the child or young person to achieve that insight, control and adjustment to his external circumstances which will enable him to return to life in the community. A family service which would involve integration of fieldwork specialities serving residential places for children would necessarily bring together these three types of provision. The Government White Paper *The Child, the Family and the Young Offender* (H.M.S.O., Cmnd. 2742) does in fact make proposals for bringing approved schools into the same system as 'other children's

71

homes'. The suggestion is made that new Family Courts should commit all children under the age of sixteen years needing placement away from home to the care of the local authority which would then decide on the type of treatment most appropriate at that stage.

It is doubtful whether this inclusion of children's homes in the category of residential places with a predominantly therapeutic approach would have been acceptable before 1948 or even in the first decade of the operation of the Children Act. The traditional function of the children's home was that of providing shelter, or in some cases and more positively, a complete substitute home. The 'village' or 'cottage' homes of the nineteenth century, many still in use today; the small 'family group homes' on housing estates which now constitute three-quarters of all local authority homes (H.M.S.O., *Report on the work of the Home Office Children's Branch 1961—1963*), are witnesses to the idea that children's homes should offer a replacement for life with the child's own parents and that they should therefore approximate to the conditions of normal family life.

Consideration was given in the last chapter to factors which have affected the development of foster care in recent years. Residential care has been similarly affected. In past years a child would remain in a children's home from the time of his admission from the nursery at the age of five years until he left to go into employment at school leaving age. Now, after a much shorter period he is likely to leave the children's home in order to return to his own parents or to be boarded out. The local authority children's home cannot be a complete substitute home, partly because the adults and children form a changing population, partly because the child cannot look ahead to his early adult years there.

The local authority children's home is therefore coming to be regarded as a therapeutic establishment; a place where children can live during periods when their needs cannot be met either in their own homes or in foster homes and where they may receive help which will enable them to return to the community.

## Reception centres, nurseries and children's homes

*The reception centre.* Section 15(2) of the Children Act 1948 states 'The accommodation provided . . . by a local authority shall include separate accommodation for the temporary reception of children, with in particular, the necessary facilities for observation of their physical and mental condition'.

Reception centres are used for the accommodation of children recently admitted to care for long or indefinite periods and for children in care who have had to leave a foster home or children's home.

The functions of these centres have not been confined, however, to the assessment of children in the care of local authorities. The Children and Young Persons (Amendment) Act 1952 empowered courts to remand children under twelve years of age, charged with or found guilty of an offence, to a special reception centre instead of to a remand home; the Children and Young Persons Act 1963 extended the age limit to fifteen years. Reception centres are also used for children who have appeared before a juvenile court as being in need of care, protection or control where the magistrates, having found the case proved, make either an interim fit person order or a place of safety order, so that various reports may be obtained before a decision is made about the future. In the case of these children, offenders or non-offenders, who are in reception centres for interim periods of three to four weeks the Superintendent of the centre, together perhaps with a psychiatrist, doctor, psychologist and teacher is usually asked to provide a report to help the magistrates to make their decision. The centre may also be used as a place of safety for children removed from their surroundings in an emergency by the police, N.S.P.C.C. or children's officer.

A reception centre is therefore dealing with children in a variety of situations: delinquents and non-delinquents, children in care and children on temporary court orders, children recently separated from their parents, and children who have been in care for some time. These children, however, have certain things in common: all of them have had a recent experience of leaving familiar surroundings, and all of them have some uncertainty about their future.

The reception centre has two main functions, to assess and to sustain. The staff have to get to know the child; to discover the ways in which he relates to them and to his family and friends, the type of behaviour he shows under stress, the extent of his social and intellectual ability, the nature of any physical handicaps or illnesses. They also have to help the child to deal with the first impact of separation and uncertainty, to make for himself a picture of the past and to look ahead to future possibilities. The centre is usually the child's first experience of being in care and it can both set the pattern of his expectations and demonstrate what may be expected of him.

*The residential nursery.* Many local authorities and voluntary societies maintain residential nurseries for children under the age of five years who cannot be boarded out.

Since 1948, however, there has been a growing appreciation of the dangers of institutionalising the pre-school child in an establishment of this kind. Some children's departments have experimented with other forms of care for babies and toddlers and have ceased to include a nursery in their residential provision. Experience shows that most of these children can be cared for successfully in small children's homes where they do not have to compete for attention with so many others of the same age group.

*The children's home.* It is not possible here, for reasons of space, to make any attempt at a classification of children's homes. A detailed description of various types of children's homes and hostels will be found in Part 2 of *Children in Homes* (Brill and Thomas, 1965). Children's homes vary in size, in staffing, in structure and in their siting. There are perhaps signs that with the abandonment of attempts to provide a complete replica of normal home life, the larger children's home may come back into favour.

## The residential worker

Changes in the function of residential care over the past twenty years have naturally resulted in changes in the role of the residential worker. In the years before 1950 the staffs of most children's homes and nurseries probably saw themselves as officials leading their lives separately from yet adjacent to the children they cared for. The development of the idea of the very small home on a housing estate involved an attempt to change their role to that of the parent substitute with a life completely merged into the 'family' group. In recent years there has been a gradual appreciation that the provision of a healing environment for a group of disturbed children demands skill and knowledge as well as qualities of personality: accordingly, there has been a new emphasis on the *professional* nature of the task. The present dilemma of residential child care is how to provide the conditions for good professional work without destroying the warm secure atmosphere of the home in which it is to be performed; how to give the individual member of staff sufficient privacy and protection from the tensions of the group and yet retain for the children a sense of 'belonging' in a homely environment.

Clare Winnicott has described the function of the residential worker in terms of the provision of good experiences of care, comfort and control which are 'not only the stuff of life, but the stuff that dreams are made of, and have the power to become part of the child's inner psychic reality, correcting the past and creating the future' (Winnicott, 1964). The houseparent provides these experiences for individual children who are living in a group. Each child will need to have a special relationship with one of the adults in the home: each adult will be concerned with meeting the different, and often competing needs of several children. The experience of a child in a children's home is not, however, only an experience of relationship with adults; relationships with other children will be of equal or greater importance. The residential worker must therefore develop skills in working with a group of children: the child care officer must not lose sight of the importance of the life of the group to 'her' child in a children's home.

*The parent and the residential worker*

The residential child care worker spends his professional

life looking after other people's children. He cares deeply about their well-being and by the fact of his appointment has received the seal of official approval on his ability to fill a parental role. In contrast, most parents of children in care feel that they have failed in many areas of their life and they have, by definition, been unsuccessful in providing continuous care for their children. It is not surprising, therefore, that their attitude towards 'the expert' who has taken over their function in this respect usually contains elements of envy, resentment and hostility. It is perhaps more remarkable that we so often expect them to feel grateful, to show unmixed pleasure in the fact that the children's home is providing better clothes and food, a more comfortable material environment, than they themselves are able to supply. The parent who neglects his children and later criticises the diet or clothing standards in the residential establishment is well known to child care workers. The criticism, the open hostility, the failure to visit or the immoderate drinking just before doing so are all ways in which mothers and fathers commonly try to deal with their fears that not only the staff, but also their own children, are judging them bad and inadequate parents.

Residential workers, unlike the parents of children in care, usually lead well organised and very busy lives. It is not easy for them to understand the muddle and confusion which result in the missed bus; or the childlike craving for immediate satisfaction which leads a father to spend his fare money on drinks and cigarettes. They see only the unhappiness of the child who waits by the window all afternoon for a visit that never happens, and they find that unhappiness difficult to bear.

The difficulties in communication and understanding

which result from these considerations are exacerbated by a lack of clarity in the role definition of the residential worker in relation to parents. The traditional division of function which regards the parent as excusively the province of the field worker, and the child as the concern of the houseparent, is unsound; since both field and residential workers are nowadays concerned in trying to heal relationships between parents and children. The residential worker has a function in relation to parents which is not solely that of saying welcoming words on visiting days. Many parents themselves have strong unsatisfied needs for parental concern and affection. They may indeed envy the experience of good care which the residential establishment is providing for their children. If they feel that they are valued by the houseparent not only as parents to the child but as people in their own right; if the housemother can provide them with food and warmth and comfort when they visit, they may perhaps be better able to accept what the establishment is offering to their child. If they do not find this acceptance, work with the child will inevitably suffer and the chances of successful rehabilitation will be remote.

The amount of participation by parents in the day to day life of the residential establishment will of course vary according to the needs of staff and children. There should perhaps in residential care be a range of provision on a continuum which has at one end the hostel accommodating whole families; and at the other the home for severely maladjusted children where parental visiting may be carefully controlled according to the degree of strain from external pressures which can be tolerated by individuals and the group. The intervening points would be occupied by homes providing various facilities for parental involvement including accommodation for weekend and holiday visits and rooms where families could spend time together in privacy. This is to some extent a new concept of residential work and one which would demand fresh skills and bring both new pressures and new satisfactions to the residential worker.

## Working with the child in residential care

No statutory provisions comparable to the Boarding Out of Children Regulations govern the visiting by child care officers of individual children in residential accommodation. The Administration of Children's Homes Regulations 1951 which specify among other things certain standards of medical care, record keeping and punishment, provide only for monthly visits by an officer or committee member in order to ascertain that the home is conducted 'in the interests of the well-being of the children'. Perhaps this absence of statutory requirement, together with an assurance that the child's physical needs are being met, account for the fact that children established in homes receive less than their share of attention from child care officers. Many feel indeed that they have no function with children in residential care except when there are arrangements to be made and plans to be discussed with the housemother. Yet the child in a children's home needs two different kinds of relationship with professional staff. He needs the residential worker who can provide the direct experiences described by Clare Winnicott (*op. cit.*) and a caseworker who can stand outside his immediate experience and hold together for him the various fragmented parts of his life.

The caseworker who saw the child with his parents, who shared with him the experience of his reception into care, or who visited him in a previous foster home will of course have a special importance for him in a children's home. The child care officer who takes on a child already placed in residential care can, however, *know about* his previous experiences and relationships, can help him to discuss them and to make them part of his present self; she can help him to talk about some of his frightened angry feelings so that they become safer and less worrying; she can enable him to remember the happy times as well as the miserable ones, his good feelings as well as his destructive wishes; she can help him to deal with some of his confused fears and fantasies about past events and his share in them. All this will involve the caseworker in sharing with the child the reality of his sadness and sense of loss, in the painful realisation that she is not able, omnipotently, to create order and happiness in his world.

### The residential worker and the child care officer

In the early years of children's departments, residential and field staff were sometimes in open conflict. Residential workers felt that the emphasis on foster care not only undervalued the work done in children's homes but also deprived them of their most rewarding children. There is now a greater degree of understanding between these two branches of the child care profession, but some difficulties still remain. These result partly from present inequalities in status and standards of training, partly from the fact that rapidly changing ideas about the function of residential care have made it hard for the residential worker to define his role. Moreover, there are the stresses in relationship which spring from the nature of the work itself and which often arise out of idealisation and envy. The child care officer, as she drives into the night, carries with her a cosy image of the housemother feeding, washing and putting to bed, and some part of her would like the satisfactions that come from these activities. The houseparent, on the other hand, sees the field worker as possessing an enviable mobility and freedom from the physical drudgery which the care of children entails. Moreover, child care officer and residential worker represent different parts of the child's life and know him in different ways; each may want to feel that their own picture is complete and yet each has to acknowledge that they both contribute to the child's reality.

# 7

# Adoption

## General

As we saw in the first chapter, public authorities in Great Britain have provided foster care and residential care for deprived children for several hundred years: adoption on the other hand became a legal procedure in England and Wales as recently as 1926, and the first Adoption Act applicable to Scotland was passed in 1930. The practice of taking a child into a private home and bringing him up as a member of the family has, however, been customary in many nationalities and among all social classes for centuries; literally, it is as old as Moses.

The Hurst Committee (H.M.S.O., 1954) appointed to consider the existing adoption law and the desirability of introducing changes in policy and procedure, gave their view of the position since the first Adoption Act of 1926. 'We are satisfied that, in spite of various shortcomings in law and administration and of the fallibility of human judgment, the general result of legalised adoption has been to increase immeasurably the happiness and well-being of probably over a million members of the community.' The report of the Hurst Committee was followed by the Adoption Act 1958, which governs current adoption practice.

Legal adoption is a process whereby

'all rights, duties, obligations and liabilities of the parents or guardians of the infant in relation to the future custody, maintenance and education of the infant . . . shall be extinguished, and all such rights, duties, obligations and liabilities shall vest in and be exercisable by and enforceable against the adoptor as if the infant were a child born to the adoptor in lawful wedlock'; (Adoption Act 1958, Section 13).

Adoption Orders may be made in England by juvenile courts, county courts, or by the High Court. An order once made is irrevocable and has equal validity whichever type of court has granted it.

Children's departments have four separate and distinct functions in adoption : they register adoption societies whose headquarters are situated within their administrative area; they may themselves act as an adoption agency; they supervise children placed for adoption by third parties and children in respect of whom notification of intention to adopt has been given; and they undertake the duties of guardian *ad litem* in adoption proceedings.

## The registration of adoption societies

A child may be placed for adoption directly by his parent or guardian; by a third party, that is, a private individual other than a parent or guardian; by a local authority or by a registered adoption agency. The large children's societies, Dr. Barnardo's, The National Children's Home, The Church of England Children's Society and the Roman Catholic children's societies are adoption agencies. There are, in addition, some sixty adoption societies in England

and Wales who are not child-caring agencies and whose work is confined to placing children in adoptive homes. Some cover the whole country, others place children within the relatively small area surrounding their office; some are non-denominational, others have a specific religious bias.

No body of persons other than a registered adoption society or local authority may make arrangements for the adoption of an infant, an 'infant' in the context of adoption law being a person under twenty-one years of age. The local authority registering an adoption agency must ascertain that it is a charitable association and may refuse registration if a reasonable number of competent staff is not employed.

## The children's committee as adoption agency

Children's committees were specifically empowered to act as adoption agencies by the 1958 Act, although some were in fact placing children other than those in care for many years before this date. In some departments the work of dealing with applications from prospective adoptors on the one hand, and parents wishing to place their children on the other, is dealt with by specialist adoption staff : in others it is included in the work of the child care officer. Some children's committees have decided not to exercise their powers of acting as an adoption placing agency because the needs of their area appear to be fully met by a local adoption society. Children's committees are necessarily non-denominational in their approach to the selection of adoptive parents, and many are prepared to consider applications from adoptors who are not regular attenders at church or chapel. The extent to which local authorities accept agnostic and atheist adoptors is governed partly by the views of the members, partly by the number of available babies whose mothers do not wish to exercise their legal right of determining that their child shall be brought up in a religious faith. Goodacre (1966) found that social class was the factor most clearly distinguishing local authority adoptors from those who had proceeded through a voluntary society. In her sample 42% of all adoptors in the two upper social classes (Registrar General's classes I and II) had proceeded through societies and only 16% had obtained their baby through the local authority. Among the two lowest classes (Registrar General's classes IV and V) the position was reversed; adoption societies were responsible for only 7% of placements with these couples and the local authority for 39%.

## Supervision of children placed for adoption

Reference was made in Chapter 5 to the provisions relating to protected children in section 37 of the Adoption Act 1958. A protected child is therein defined as:

(a) a child below the upper limit of compulsory school age who is placed in the care and possession of a person who is not a parent, guardian or relative of his and another person, not being a parent or guardian of his, takes part in the arrangements; and

(b) a child in respect of whom notice of intention to apply for an adoption order has been given.

Under (a) children's departments have duties towards all children who are placed for adoption by third parties. The third party may be a relation, the matron of a maternity home, a general practitioner, a neighbour or any person willing to act as a go-between who knows of a baby in need of a home and a couple who want a child. The percentage of all adoptions arranged by third parties is not known. Goodacre (1966) found that they accounted for only 3% of the placements in her sample and a recent unpublished pilot study of court records undertaken by the Home Office Research Unit, in conjunction with the Government Social Survey, would support the view that the proportion involved is small. Although there is no research evidence about the comparative success of different methods of placement in this country, the experience of many children's departments suggests that this small number of third party placements accounts for a high proportion of the unsatisfactory adoptions. It is known that many couples whose applications have been refused by adoption agencies find babies in this way. The Hurst Committee accepted that individuals acting as third parties usually lack the skills and qualifications necessary for their task and frequently consider the interests of adoptors or the natural mother rather than those of the child. Nevertheless, they decided that the prohibition of such placements would not be wise or practicable. The 1958 Adoption Act provides that third parties must notify the local authority fourteen days before placing a child in order that the children's department may satisfy themselves that the home is not unsuitable. In practice this requirement is often evaded through the claim that the arrangement was made in an emergency when the statutory notification can be delayed until up to a week after placement. The local authority can prohibit the placing of a child in a home if it appears that it would be detrimental to him to be kept by that person in those premises, but even the full fourteen days' notice allows only a superficial investigation of the home. In these situations the child care officer is usually regarded at first as an unwelcome inspector with power to prevent the fulfilment of arranged plans. If, however, she is aware of the anxiety and need lying behind any hostility in the prospective adoptors, her recognition of this may do much to dispel it.

Under (b) of section 37 of the Adoption Act 1958, a child also becomes 'protected' if notice of intention to apply for an adoption order has been given in respect of him. The Act provides that except where one of the applicants is a parent of the child, an adoption order shall not be made by a court in respect of an infant of school age or under unless three months before the date of the order the applicant has given notice in writing to the appropriate local authority of his intention to apply to a court for an adoption order. The children's department then has a duty to satisfy itself of the well-being of the child by means of visits, and this responsibility continues until the adoption order is made or he reaches the age of eighteen years.

Many child care officers are uncertain of their function during this period of 'welfare supervision', particularly if the child has been placed by an adoption agency when the infant's physical well-being and the material conditions of the home normally give no grounds for anxiety.

The child care officer's uncertainty about her functions is usually shared by the adoptive parents. These have, at least in the case of adoption agency placements, already undergone searching enquiries relating both to their circumstances and their attitudes. They have often formed a relationship of confidence with the agency worker who, in many instances, will continue to visit until the order is made. The investigations by the representative of the Court loom ahead, and apprehension about these proceedings, together with fears that the mother will not finally give her consent, often occupy the forefront of their minds. In the meantime they must, in the case of a first adoption, accustom themselves to new roles and unfamiliar feelings. Some of these will be common to all new parents: the relationship between husband and wife will change subtly as the wife becomes preoccupied with her maternal role; the anxiety about the physical care of a small infant will impose strains on both of them; there will be a new balance in their relationships with neighbours and the wider family. In addition to these adjustments, adoptors will experience for the first time the strong emotions aroused by this baby born of other parents: they may find that he stirs unresolved sorrow about their own childlessness, and that they have unsuspected feelings about the child's own mother and father. They may too have half-acknowledged worries about their ability to love him as they would a child of their own. Into this complicated situation comes the child care officer; a stranger who has undefined powers and whose opinion of them and of their home may affect the success of the application for an adoption order.

In such a situation of uncertainty on both sides, it is not surprising that many adoption supervision visits turn into social occasions during which the child care officer makes reassuring and admiring remarks about the baby and the adoptors offer uncertain cups of tea and comments about the weather.

The case for combining the duties of welfare supervision with those of the guardian *ad litem*, the officer of the court, in all but privately arranged adoptions, could perhaps be maintained on the grounds that adoptors should not be subjected to intimate enquiries from three separate officials during this period in their lives. However, it is clear that some adoptors can be helped to use welfare supervision constructively. The child care officer may in fact be the only person to whom they feel they can safely confide uncertainties and anxieties. To their neighbours and families they must firmly assert that everything is perfect; the adoption agency did, after all, provide the baby; the guardian *ad litem* has too much of the aura of the law. The child care officer coming into the situation at the point of stress may sometimes help adoptors to voice and face their doubts and worries, their guilt at having someone's else's baby, their concern about whether their feelings in this situation are 'normal' and acceptable. The child care officer must try to recognise the adoptors who need this help; she must equally respect the defences of those who cannot make use of it at this time.

## The duties of guardian ad litem

In any application for an adoption order in England the Court must appoint some person to act as 'Guardian *ad litem* of the infant', with the duty of safeguarding the interests of the infant before the court. This function is normally undertaken by a probation officer or the children's officer in juvenile and county courts, and by the official solicitor in the High Court. The duties of the guardian *ad litem* are specified in the Adoption Rules. Broadly, these are to investigate the circumstances of the adoption, to ascertain the physical and economic state of the applicants and their home, to interview all the people concerned, including the natural parents and anyone involved in arranging the placement, and to make sure that all the necessary consents have been freely given. The

89

guardian *ad litem* must also decide whether the 'infant' is able to understand the nature of an adoption order and if so, whether he wishes to be adopted by the applicants; a requirement which may present problems, since children can understand the meaning of adoption at different levels and at different ages, according to their stage of development.

The guardian *ad litem* has an onerous task, since besides checking facts and considering legal detail, he has to make an assessment of relationships and attitudes in the adoptive home to help the Court to decide whether an order will be for the welfare of the child. Where the children's officer is appointed as guardian *ad litem*, the duties may be performed by a specialist officer or may be included in the normal work of the child care officer. In the latter case the same person may be responsible for visiting the adoptive home for the purposes of both welfare supervision and guardian *ad litem*. Where the children's department has itself acted as adoption agency the court usually appoints a probation officer to act as guardian *ad litem*.

*The selection of children for adoption*

Adoption agencies usually try to form some estimate of an infant's likely inheritance of mental and physical health from a detailed examination of the family background of both parents. The present state of our knowledge about genetics, however, severely limits the accuracy of any such forecast. A detailed report on the child's health must be obtained by the agency before the adoption placement and in addition, the court dealing with the application for an order requires a full medical report on the child concerned. There are no absolute standards of good heredity or physical and mental fitness required by law of an adopted child. The courts are only concerned that adoptors shall understand and accept all the known risks to the future health of the infant: if these are serious the court would need some assurance that the adoptors could cope with any resulting difficulties. A child can therefore be adopted if adoptors can be found who are willing and suitable to adopt him. There are no children who are inherently unadoptable.

Some adoption agencies have strict rules of their own about the categories of children they will not accept for placement: those born as a result of a second illegitimate pregnancy, for instance, or legitimate offspring of a marriage. Local authorities may be more disposed than the specialist societies to see adoption as one of several methods of providing for the upbringing of the child and consequently to consider what arrangements they will be able to make for his future if he is not placed with adoptive parents.

*Adoptive parents*

It is not possible in a work of this size to give detailed consideration to criteria for the selection of adoptive parents. As with the infants themselves, some agencies have fixed rules about the eligibility of couples for consideration. The age and marital status of prospective adoptors; the duration of the marriage; the presence or absence of natural children of the marriage; the degree of certainty about fertility; the level of income, employment security and religious allegiance, are all factors which are taken into account, although agencies differ in opinion about their significance. There is as yet little research evidence about the characteristics of the successful adoptive home, but on some points perhaps there is a consensus of opinion among workers in the field. It seems likely that the most successful adoptive parents are those who are able to face the realities of the adoptive situation. If they are childless this will imply that they have achieved some degree of acceptance of their inability to produce children : if they already have a child or children of their own, that they have the ability to come to terms with the difference between natural and adoptive parenthood. Kirk (1964) has described in sociological terms the 'role handicap' of adoptive parents in a society where biological parenthood is the norm, and concludes that their capacity for bearing the pain involved in the 'acknowledgment of difference' is crucial to the success of the adoption. In this connection the attitude of adoptors to the natural parents of the child has great importance. Some adoptors try to deal with their guilt about acting as parents to a child who was not born to them by seeing the biological mother as bad and adoption as a rescue operation. Other adoptors may try to deny the existence of the natural mother by shared fantasies that the child is their own or, more commonly, by vehemently asserting the irrelevance of genetic factors in the formation of physique and personality.

Considerable publicity has been given to the opinion of most adoption workers that children should be told of their adoption at an early age. Accordingly, most prospective adoptors will volunteer their readiness to do this. It is not, however, a once-for-all process and cannot be achieved by a single story about the much-wanted baby told to a three-year-old child. Many adoptors find even this initial stage hard to bear and discussions stretching on into adolescence and beyond which involve giving some picture of the natural mother and father present greater difficulties. Adoptive parents do not have an easy task. They must fully commit themselves to the child and love him as their own, yet they must be prepared to face with him the fact that he was born to other parents. McWhinnie (1967) in her study of adopted children in adult life has illustrated the problems of communication in this area between children and adoptive parents.

## Natural parents

In this chapter little has been written about the natural parents of adopted children. The need of the mothers for casework help during the time when they are deciding about their baby's future, at the time of separation if the child is placed for adoption, and during the subsequent periods of mourning and readjustment need not be emphasised. That the fathers of illegitimate babies also require help is only just beginning to receive recognition. In some authorities the children's department provides a casework service for unmarried parents; in others this work is undertaken by a moral welfare association. Adoption is, of course, not the only possibility open to the unmarried mother: it seems clear that more unmarried mothers would keep their children if there were a more accepting public attitude and more long-term services to help them.

## Further considerations

From one viewpoint adoption, along with residential care and boarding out, is a method of providing for children who are unable to live with their natural parents. Until recently it has nevertheless been set apart from other child care services and it has tended to attract different social attitudes. Adopted children were perhaps in some ways regarded as the aristocracy of the deprived, the label 'suitable for adoption' implying a guarantee of physical and mental quality: to be 'unadoptable' has meant that someone must be paid to look after you. Adoptive parents have received a social approval not experienced by foster mothers who, perhaps by reason of their acceptance of boarding out allowances, have had in the minds of many people a faint aura of the nineteenth century baby farmer. Adoption in fact has suffered neither the taint of the Poor Law which local authority child care is only now beginning to dispel, nor the aroma of Victorian charity from which the voluntary children's societies have suffered. This is perhaps partly because the need to provide for the care of an illegitimate infant is known in the most illustrious circles and the longing of childless couples for a baby of their own is not confined to one social class.

These considerations may have some bearing on three interesting points about adoption. Firstly, the decision to accept a couple as adoptive parents and to place a baby with them is as far reaching in its effects as any which social workers have to make. Yet it is only very recently that adoption has come to be regarded as a field in which trained caseworkers are essential. Social work attention has in this country been traditionally regarded as the prerogative of the lowest socio-economic groups, and adoptors are not normally drawn from this section of the community. Secondly, when in the field of child care as a whole, emphasis is increasingly placed on helping children and those who care for them to accept the realities of the situation, when the need for children to have knowledge about their natural parents as real people is accepted, an atmosphere of secrecy still surrounds adoption. An adopted child has little power to obtain information about his origins and many are given only the sketchiest picture of their parents and wider family. Thirdly, when much modern psychological thinking underlines the importance of continuous care for even small infants, babies sometimes have a succession of temporary placements before going to their adoptive home, partly in order to avoid subjecting adoptors to the stress of uncertain maternal decisions. It is clear that many mothers need time after their confinement in order to make an unhurried decision about their own future and that of the baby. It is also undeniable that stress in the adoptive mother may adversely affect her handling of the infant. The problem of the age at which a baby should be placed for adoption must be considered afresh in each individual case : it does not admit of any easy answer, since it often involves real conflicts of interest between the parties involved. In this situation, however, the baby is the most vulnerable client and the greatest weight has to be given to his needs.

# 8

# The children's department

## Relationship with the community

As the foregoing chapters have shown, children's departments are organisations concerned with meeting some of the needs of children and of families within their administrative area. But they are not independent entities. A children's department derives its resources and its sanctions from the social environment; it is also itself one of the forces which affect and mould the attitudes of society towards those who need its help. This chapter considers firstly some of the ways in which a children's department interacts with society, and secondly the place of the social worker within the organisation.

Communication between a children's department and the general public is carried out formally and informally at many different levels. A Member of Parliament asks a question in the House about the treatment of a child in a foster home; an assistant housemother talks about her work while buying the groceries; there are comments in the local press about the siting of a proposed children's home; a child care officer addresses a meeting of the Women's Institute; a children's committee member receives letters of protest about the closing down of a family advice centre. The treatment of juvenile delinquents in approved schools, the care of deprived children, the inadequacies of 'problem families' are all matters which arouse considerable public interest and emotion and are the subjects of strongly held views amongst the electorate. The two-way process of communication between the child care service and the community is itself one of the factors responsible for gradual changes in public attitudes and these changes enable new provision to be made. It is, for instance, very doubtful whether the powers given local authorities by section 1 of the Children and Young Persons Act of 1963 would have been acceptable to the general public fifteen years before: since 1948 the community has been moving towards an acceptance of the idea that some of its members, among them parents of families, are socially handicapped and need assistance which goes beyond the bounds of equitable treatment.

The electorate provides for and controls the child care service through the machinery of central and local government; through Parliament and the Home Office, and through county and county borough councils.

## Parliament and the Home Office

Parliamentary legislation sets the broad limits of the work of a children's department and defines its powers and duties. The Secretary of State for the Home Office, the Minister with parliamentary responsibility for the service, is empowered to make detailed regulations relating to the way in which departments carry out certain aspects of their work and these regulations are legally binding: examples are the Boarding Out Regulations and the Adoption Agency Regulations to which reference has already been made.

The Home Office, through its Inspectorate, provides a service of consultation to departments and seeks to ensure that they are fulfilling their statutory obligations and are maintaining acceptable standards. The Home Secretary appoints two standing councils, representative of informed opinion, to advise him on matters connected with the child care service: the Advisory Council on Child Care and the Central Training Council. He will also seek the advice of the Local Authority Associations before introducing any important legal or administrative changes.

Central government is concerned with the finances of the child care service and meets part of the cost. Certain functions under the Children Act 1948 were among those in respect of which the general grant under the Local Government Act 1958 replaced the old percentage grants: if a local authority does not maintain a reasonable standard in the provision of child care services therefore, Parliament may reduce its general grant. In addition, broadly 50% of approved expenditure on the maintenance of remand homes and approved schools is met by a specific grant. Moreover, if a local authority needs to borrow money to build or to acquire land, sanction for the loan must be given by the Ministry of Housing and Local Government: if the project were, for instance, a children's home this Ministry would require an assurance from the Home Office that the plans met with their approval.

In these ways the nation, through its parliamentary electorate and central government departments, exercises a control over child care provision. It is perhaps fortunate that child care is not one of the subjects which has so far attracted political alignments in Parliament, but nevertheless Members interest themselves in the work and from time to time ask questions in and out of the House about both policy and specific cases. Such questions are normally addressed to the Home Secretary who always gets the observations of the local authority concerned before attempting a reply.

## Local government; the council and the children's committee

There is a legal obligation on county borough, county and London borough councils (unless the Home Secretary otherwise directs) to appoint a children's committee for the purpose of functions under the Children and Young Persons Acts, the Children Acts and the Adoption Act. The children's committee (as the welfare, education and fire brigade committees, amongst others) is thus one of the statutory local government committees to which matters relating to certain specified functions stand referred. A local government committee may not raise a rate nor borrow money. These powers are the prerogative of the main council, which is responsible for allocating the financial resources of the authority between its spending committees. Children's committees normally submit estimates of their expenditure during the forthcoming financial year to the finance committee, whose recommendations are in turn considered by a meeting of the council in the light of their total estimated outlay and income. The financial resources of a children's department are therefore controlled directly by the representatives of the community in which it works, and in the case of certain expenditure further control is exercised by central government departments and ultimately by Parliament.

A council may decide to delegate nearly all its powers to its various committees and the scheme of delegation is set out in the standing orders of each local authority. A children's committee may thus be empowered to spend sums of a certain magnitude on projects within its approved estimate provision without the further approval of the council, but will have to seek this approval for other developments involving large sums of money. The main children's committee may, in its turn, delegate the power to decide on expenditure within defined limits to one of its sub-committees or to the children's officer. The exact pattern will show considerable variation between one authority and another. In one area, for instance, a holiday grant of £20 for a foster child may require approval from the full children's committee; in another, the area or case committee will give final approval; and in a third, the children's officer may be empowered to act without reference to any committee. The children's officer may of course allow his power of making this kind of decision to be exercised by one of his senior staff.

The composition of the children's committee is laid down in the Children Act 1948. It may include co-opted members—persons specially qualified by reason of experience or training—but elected members of the council must be in the majority. The size of the children's committee varies from one authority to another as do the number and the organisation of the sub-committees to which the main committee may delegate its functions. Again, the Children Act provides that each sub-committee must include at least one member of the local authority. In a large county or county borough the main children's committee will probably confine itself to broad issues of policy and all the detailed work will be carried out by sub-committees, whereas in a small authority the members of the children's committee may well know all the staff of the department and the circumstances of most of the children in care.

The children's committee then, is responsible for the functions delegated to it by the council and for the general work of the department. The council will receive periodic reports from the committee, will ratify its decisions where necessary, and will decide on the basis of the estimates it provides how much money to allocate to the child care service.

Within broad limits, therefore, the amount of money an authority spends on its children's service bears some relation to the ability of children's committee members to convince the main council of the importance of the work. The annual sum spent is of course affected by local needs, circumstances and costs, as well as by council attitudes. That there are wide variations is shown by the fact that in 1965–66 Oldham spent on the child care service more than ten times, and Blackpool less than twice, the product of a penny rate (Institute of Municipal Treasurers, 1966).

*Professional child care worker and committee member*

The relationship between local government officers and members of local authorities and committees is not easy to describe in detail. In general, the officer is the servant of the council whose function is 'to advise and to carry out the lawful instructions of his local authority, and to exercise on their behalf such functions as have been delegated to him' (Jackson, 1966). The extent to which committees give instructions about the day to day work of the officer varies. In larger authorities, as we have seen, the children's committee is mainly concerned with policy and financial matters and there is considerable delegation, not only to subcommittees, but also to the children's officer. In other authorities committees enter into decisions about the approval of foster homes or the future of individual children.

There is some divergence of views about the extent to which the lay committee should concern themselves with the details of departmental work: this applies not only in the field of child care but over the whole area of local government. The recent reports of both the Maud (H.M.S.O., 1967a) and Mallaby (H.M.S.O., 1967b) Committees suggest that local authorities should entrust greater responsibilities to their officers so that the more efficient conduct of business would be facilitated by ensuring that decisions are taken at the appropriate level.

The local government officer with professional training is a servant of his employing authority no less than his administrative and clerical colleagues, but he also has an allegiance to the standards and values of his profession. If he is at issue with the council which employs him over a matter in which he has professional competence he has a right to offer advice and may thereby seek to change their views; ultimately he may decide that he cannot continue in their service. He has, it is clear (except in certain very limited functions), no right to act in contradiction of their instructions whether he be doctor, solicitor or engineer. These are, however, old established professions and the lay committee member might well hesitate to invade the domain of their knowledge. On the other hand, the member as a parent may consider his judgment of a child care issue to be as valid as that of the trained or experienced social worker.

It is perhaps this lack of clear agreement about the area of their professional competence, together with fears about the safety of confidential information, which makes many children's officers reluctant to tell committees more than is absolutely necessary about the work of their departments.

This attitude is understandable in view of the potentially damaging results to children of unwise committee decisions or of details about the private lives of clients becoming known in their neighbourhood.

The case for reporting fully to committees about the work of a department, however can be substantiated on five counts.

Firstly, the children's committee has, under the council, final responsibility for the work done by its child care staff. Those who are engaged in child care, whether as administrators, residential works or field workers are highly vulnerable to public opinion and public displeasure, and they need the support of the representatives of society. It is therefore proper for a committee to be asked to decide on behalf of the community whether, for instance, a child should be placed with a foster father who has committed a criminal offence. The child care officer has the serious responsibility in this case of deciding what advice to offer to the committee; the final decision must be that of the committee alone, because if anything goes wrong as a result of the child's placement in the home, the public will call it to account. In this connection the report of the Chief Inspector on the inspection of the Dorset County Council Child Care Service (H.M.S.O., 1966c) emphasises the importance of informing the children's committee of matters seriously affecting the welfare of a child in care.

Secondly, the committee obtains and controls the resources of the department and makes important decisions about policy and provision. In local government as a whole, and in the child care service in particular, policy is not a body of theoretical guide lines to action; it is intimately bound up with the well-being of individuals. If committees are not given the means of understanding the

103

real problems and needs of those for whom they provide the service it is not easy for them to make wise policy decisions or to allocate resources prudently.

Thirdly, the committee must keep the practice of the professional worker in line with what society will accept. This aspect of their function is particularly important at the present time when social attitudes towards human relationships and behaviour are changing rapidly. The child care worker looking closely at the needs of a child in care or a family with problems must also be aware of the feelings and interests of the community in which they live. The need to justify before a lay committee the advisability of a certain course of action not only ensures some clarification of plans and objectives, but also prevents the child care officer from becoming out of touch with the demands which society may make on his clients.

Further, the committee is itself an educative force in society. A real understanding by members of the needs of the department's clients is likely to have repercussions on social policy and attitudes because those engaged in local government frequently have wide contacts and hold membership of other committees and bodies. The complaint that society does not understand the problems of the child in care or the multi-problem family is often made by those who would deny members of children's committees the opportunity of feeling their way into these problems through knowledge about individual cases. It is no part of the committee member's function to have personal contact with clients, but through the child care officer he can be helped to apprehend some of the difficulties faced by them.

Lastly, the relationship of child care worker to committees and their members must be based on an understanding

THE CHILDREN'S DEPARTMENT

of each other's proper function and a mutual respect and confidence. The child care officer must feel she can rely on the discretion of individual members and on the weight of judgment in the committee: members must be able to trust the officer's professional knowledge and recommendations. The image of social workers has suffered because of their inability to communicate to those outside their work what they are trying to achieve and the means by which they seek to achieve it. A committee with real understanding of the problems facing child care staff and the way in which they deal with them tends to have increased respect for their professional competence.

## The children's officer

The structure of children's departments varies in complexity according to their size and the extent of the geographical area which they cover. All have a children's officer at the apex although in certain very small authorities the children's officer may be shared with a neighbouring authority. Under the Children Act 1948 the appointment is statutory. Provision is made for the Secretary of State to prohibit the selection of anyone whose experience and qualifications he considers inadequate, although the Maud Committee has recently recommended that the Home Secretary should cease to have this power. If the children's department is seen as an enterprise in terms of the model formulated by A. K. Rice (1963) then the children's officer is its leader who must manage the relations between the enterprise and its environment, define its primary task and keep under review both definition and constraints; he must also recruit the necessary resources for performance and control their use. Thus children's officers usually devote much of their time to committee work, to discussions with senior officers in other departments of their own authority, and to maintaining satisfactory relations with external voluntary and statutory agencies.

The responsibility of children's officers for the recruiting and control of resources is particularly important at the present time, when there are pressures on the service to take on an ever increasing volume of work, and when the resources that are limited are not only those of money but also of trained staff. The Mallaby Committee quotes the figure of 12.5% of a total of 2,675 established posts for child care officers in local authorities' children's departments as vacant on 31st March 1966: the Committee found that, in a sample of local authorities, 43.6% of child care officers possessed qualifications which were rated as less than desirable by the authority employing them (H.M.S.O., 1967b). The children's officer, therefore, frequently has to consider the needs of prospective clients which will be unmet if the department does not offer help and weigh these against the needs of those with whom his agency is already working. For example, if tenants in a given authority are in arrears with their rent and are not offered casework help by the children's department, there is a danger of some families becoming homeless and of children entering Part III Accommodation and, ultimately perhaps, being received into care. The existing team of child care officers can, however, only add to their caseloads by giving less attention to the needs of children in children's homes or by devoting less time to the recruitment and assessment of foster parents. If, on the other hand, the decision to take on this other group of clients is accompanied by an expansion in the staff establishment, the national shortage of trained staff means that inexperienced, unskilled applicants will probably fill the newly created posts. Thus, the overall standard of work is again likely to fall. This situation may perhaps be ameliorated by the more economic use of the trained caseworkers: perhaps an increase in the numbers of clerical or administrative workers would make it possible to relieve them of some functions and allow them either to take on more cases or to give additional supervision to the untrained recruits. Perhaps, on the other hand, an increase in residential provision would obviate the need for time-consuming short-term foster placements, yet provide equally satisfactory experiences for the children concerned.

The children's officer has to be constantly reviewing the objectives and priorities of his department, and in the light of this activity must make decisions about the allocation of resources between the different parts of the organisation.

*Senior staff*

The extent to which other levels of management are interposed between the children's officer and the child care officer will depend on the size of the department. In some there is a range, including deputy children's officer, assistant children's officers, area officers, senior child care officers: in other very small authorities the children's officer may share the departmental caseload with one child care officer. Where there are intervening levels, however, these members of staff will be occupied to a great extent in the co-ordination of work and allocation of resources. The child care officer's work consists largely in meeting the needs of an individual child or family: the senior staff will perhaps help her to use her own resources of time and skill to recognise and meet these needs, but they will also be concerned with the conflicting demands of the child or group of children and clients on the scarce available resources of staff, building or money. They will have to consider whether Tommy Smith or John Brown has the greater need for the one vacant place in a children's home; whether the child care officer should take on her caseload this unmarried mother or that family in rent arrears; whether a grant should be given for Mrs. Jones' electricity bill; whether the area office and the clients in the south of the city have a greater need than those in the north for the services of the newly appointed child care officer.

There will also in most departments be senior staff concerned with the acquisition, budgeting and disbursement of financial resources; the fabric and equipment of children's homes; the recruitment and selection of staff; the channels of communication within the agency and between the department and the outside world. The extent to which these functions are carried out by officers with a child care or administrative background varies between authorities. The role of the specialist local government administrator in a department staffed largely by members of another profession is too large a question to be considered here. Conflicts can, and do, arise between child care and administrative staff, whether or not the administrators have a professional social work background. The conflict is often a reflection of the age-old tension between the one and the many; the child care officer seeing individual need, the administrator the demands of other clients and the claims of consistency and fairness.

*The child care officer*

In the foregoing pages the child care officer has been seen in her relationships with a wide range of people, with children and their parents, foster parents, residential workers, adoptive parents, other social workers, committee members and the hierarchy of her own department. She meets these people as a caseworker with certain legally defined responsibilities working within the administrative framework of local government. Her sanctions are those given by society in various of its organised forms to the agency that employs her. If, in the last resort, she disagrees fundamentally with the attitudes of her committee towards those clients for whom she has a professional responsibility, then she cannot continue in their employment. For although the social worker has a commitment to the unique value of each individual, it is as Halmos (1965) has illustrated, a fiction that she practices the ideal of 'total non-directiveness', and because of her local government setting, she is very closely affected by the values of society. If, for instance, she believes that young adolescent girls should receive information on birth control and be permitted to behave promiscuously, it would very difficult for her to work in an area where both the committee and public opinion hold firmly to the ideal of chastity.

The child care officer has a particular responsibility to guard the client from being treated solely on a basis of administrative convenience and expediency. In the child care service where the state is entering into very intimate areas of family relationships, the professional standing and standards of the social worker are an important safeguard of individual liberty. Within her own service, therefore, and in the variety of her relationships with the community, the child care officer must be the advocate of the needs of the individual child and family. By giving impetus to the upward flow of information about inadequate provision she can have an important effect on both local and national policy making.

The child care officer frequently stands at a point of stress and divergent interest: between the family with multiple problems and the housing committee; foster parent and adolescent girl; natural parent and adoptive parent; the family and the teenager who is out of control. There are also less obvious conflicts: between the need to act quickly and the longing for more time in which to gather information and reflect upon it; between the desire for order and the reality of messiness and confusion; between knowledge of the ideal and the necessary acceptance of second best. In these conflicts the child care officer needs the support of the structured setting in which she works and it is important that this is organised so as to provide it.

Stress and conflict are inescapable realities in the professional life of a child care officer, but the rewards and satisfactions, if intangible, are no less real. It is today unfashionable to admit to a desire to do good, and the label 'do-gooder' is regarded as pejorative by professional social workers. This is perhaps because we now recognise that what the doer regards as good does not always appear good to the recipient. Similarly, the word 'vocation' has for many become suspect and carries connotations of old-fashioned piety and untrained enthusiasm. It is thus difficult to delineate the satisfactions of the child care officer's work without sounding sentimental and out of date. For these satisfactions which touch the whole of her personality do bear some relation to a wish to do good and to help other people. They are not to be described in terms of the achievement of solid results: the real effects of social casework are difficult to measure and can rarely be regarded with the justifiable pride appropriate to the businessman viewing his trade figures, or the surgeon completing a successful operation. The child care officer's rewards have to do with the satisfaction of her own needs to nurture and protect; with her professional involvement in the growth and development of children and of families; with her opportunities for feeling with individuals at points of crisis and bewilderment; with her belief that she can offer in these situations something from herself which may help to heal relationships, to make the uncertainties safer; with her sense of reaching out to and recognising herself in the wide range of people who are her clients.

# Suggestions for further reading

This book has covered in a very condensed form a wide range of subjects within the general area of the work of a children's department. Some indications for further reading on specific points have been included in earlier chapters, others are given in the bibliography. The suggestions which follow are of books and articles which should be of particular interest to the student beginning in this branch of the social services.

FERARD, M. L. & HUNNYBUNN, K. *The Caseworker's Use of Relationships* (London : Tavistock Publications, 1962) is an interesting and readable discussion of the general principles of casework.

TIMMS, N. *Casework in the Child Care Service* (London : Butterworths, 1962) shows the application of these principles to child care and discusses in detail the work of the child care officer with foster parents, natural parents, adolescents and young children.

HEYWOOD, J. S. *Children in Care* (London : Routledge and Kegan Paul, 1959) is a history of the development of the child care services in this country from medieval times until the middle of the twentieth century.

JEHU, D. *Casework before Admission to Care* (London : Association of Child Care Officers, 1963) and STEVENSON, O. 'Reception into Care', *Case Conference*, Vol. X, No. 4, 1963, are two short articles which describe the processes involved in receiving a child into care, and examine the feelings and needs of the different people in the situation.

WINNICOTT, C. *Child Care and Social Work* (London : Codicote Press, 1964) is an invaluable collection of papers including articles on communication with children; the role of the residential child care worker; and the relationship between fieldworker and residential worker.

ROWE, J. *Parents, Children and Adoption* (London: Routledge and Kegan Paul, 1966) is recommended as a comprehensive, descriptive study of adoption in its legal, administrative and casework aspects.

WARHAM, J. *An Introduction to Administration for Social Workers* (London: Routledge and Kegan Paul, 1967) includes an outline of current theories about organisation and management and a discussion of processes of administration in social work agencies. Many of the illustrations are taken from child care.

STEVENSON, O. *An Approach to Family Social Work* (London: Routledge and Kegan Paul, 1968) and BEEDELL, C. *Residential Life with Children* (London: Routledge and Kegan Paul, 1968) are two volumes in the Library of Social Work series which are of special relevance to the work of children's departments.

The four autobiographical works at the end of the Bibliography are of value because they succeed in conveying to the reader what being in care feels like to the child concerned.

# Bibliography

BALBERNIE, R. (1966) *Residential Work with Children*, London : Pergamon Press.

BEEDELL, C. J. (1963) 'Life in Children's Homes and Staffing Policy', *Proceedings of Fourteenth Annual Conference*, Association of Children's Officers.

BEEDELL, C. J. (1968) *Residential Life with Children*, London : Routledge and Kegan Paul.

BIESTEK, F. P. (1961) *The Casework Relationship*, London : Allen & Unwin.

BOWLBY, J. (1951) *Maternal Care and Mental Health*, Geneva : World Health Organisation.

BOWLBY, J. (1953) *Child Care and the Growth of Love*, London : Penguin Books.

BRILL, K. & THOMAS, R. (1964) *Children in Homes*, London : Gollancz.

CHALONER, L. (1963) *Feeling and Perception in Young Children*, London : Tavistock Publications.

DINNAGE, R. & PRINGLE, M. L. (1967) *Residential Child Care— Facts and Fallacies*, London : Longmans, Green & Co.

DINNAGE, R. & PRINGLE, M. L. (1967) *Foster Home Care—Facts and Fallacies*, London : Longmans, Green & Co.

DONNISON, D. V. (1965) *Social Policy and Administration*, London : Allen & Unwin.

FERARD, M. L. & HUNNYBUN, N. K. (1962) *The Caseworker's Use of Relationships*, London : Tavistock Publications.

FORDER, A. (1966) *Social Casework and Administration*, London : Faber & Faber.

FRAIBERG, S. (1959) *The Magic Years*, New York : Charles Scribner.

BIBLIOGRAPHY

GOODACRE, I. (1966) *Adoption Policy and Practice*, London: Allen & Unwin.

GRAY, P. G. & PARR, E. A. (1957) 'Children in Care and the Recruitment of Foster Parents', *Social Survey*, London: H.M.S.O.

HALMOS, P. (1965) *The Faith of the Counsellors*, London: Constable & Co.

HEINICKE, C. M. & WESTHEIMER, I. J. (1955) *Brief Separations*, London: Longmans, Green & Co.

HEYWOOD, J. S. (1959) *Children in Care*, London: Routledge and Kegan Paul.

H.M.S.O. (1946) *Report of the Care of Children Committee (Curtis Report)*, Cmnd. 6922.

(1952) *Select Committee on Estimates, Sixth Report . . . Session 1951* (H.C.P. 235).

(1954) *Report of the Departmental Committee on the Adoption of Children (Hurst Report)* Cmnd. 9248.

(1960) *Report of the Committee on Children and Young Persons (Ingleby Report)* Cmnd. 1191.

(1965) *The Family, the Child and the Young Offender*, Cmnd. 2742.

(1966a) *Children in Care in England and Wales*, Cmnd. 3204.

(1966b) *Summary of Local Authorities' return of particulars of children in care at 31st March 1966.*

(1966c) *The Dorset County Council Child Care Service.*

(1967a) *Report of the Committee on Management of Local Government (Maud Report).*

(1967b) *Report of the Committee on the Staffing of Local Government (Mallaby Report).*

*Report of the Children's Branch* (various dates).

INSTITUTE OF MUNICIPAL TREASURERS AND ACCOUNTANTS, THE SOCIETY OF COUNTY TREASURERS (1966) *Children's Services Statistics, 1965—66*, London: I.M.T.

JACKSON, W. E. (1966) *The Structure of Local Government in England and Wales*, London: Longmans, Green & Co.

JEHU, D. (1963) *Casework, before admission to care*, London: Association of Child Care Officers.

KIRK, H. DAVID (1964) *Shared Fate*, New York: Free Press of Glencoe.

LEONARD, P. (1966) *Sociology in Social Work*, London: Routledge and Kegan Paul.

MCWHINNIE, A. M. (1967) *Adopted Children, How They Grow Up*, London: Routledge and Kegan Paul.

PACKMAN, J. (1968) *Child Care: Needs and Numbers*, London: Allen & Unwin.

PARKER, R. A. (1966) *Decision in Child Care*, London: Allen & Unwin.

PHILP, A. F. (1963) *Family Failure*, London: Faber & Faber.

PHILP, A. F. & TIMMS, N. *The Problems of the Problem Family*, London: Family Service Units.

PRINGLE, M. L. KELLMER. (1967) *Adoption, Facts and Fallacies*, London: Longmans, Green & Co.

RICE, A. K. (1963) *The Enterprise and its Environment*, London: Tavistock Publications.

ROWE, J. (1966) *Parents, Children and Adoption*, London: Routledge and Kegan Paul.

STEVENSON, O. (1963a) 'Co-ordination Reviewed', *Case Conference*, Vol. IX, No. 8, Feb. 1963.

(1963b) 'The Understanding Caseworker', *New Society*, 1st August 1963.

(1963c) 'Reception into Care', *Case Conference*, Vol. X, No. 4, Sept. 1963.

(1965) *Someone Else's Child, a book for foster parents of young children*, London: Routledge and Kegan Paul.

(1968) *An Approach to Family Social Work*, London: Routledge and Kegan Paul.

TOD, R. J. ed. (1968) *Papers on Residential Work: Volume I— Children in Care*, London: Longmans, Green & Co.

TOD, R. J. ed. (1968) *Papers on Residential Work: Volume II— Deprived Children*, London: Longmans, Green & Co.

TIMMS, N. (1962) *Casework in the Child Care Service*, London: Butterworths.

TRASLER, G. (1960) *In Place of Parents*, London: Routledge and Kegan Paul.

BIBLIOGRAPHY

WARHAM, J. (1967) *An Introduction to Administration to Social Workers*, London: Routledge and Kegan Paul.

WEINSTEIN, E. A. (1960) *The Self-Image of the Foster Child*, London: Russell Sage Foundation.

WILLIAMS, G. (1967) *Caring for People*, London: Allen & Unwin.

WILSON, H. (1962) *Delinquency and Child Neglect*, London: Allen & Unwin.

WIMPERIS, V. (1960) *The Unmarried Mother and her Child*, London: Allen & Unwin.

WINNICOTT, C. (1964) *Child Care and Social Work*, London: Codicote Press.

WINNICOTT, D. W. (1957) *The Child and the Family*, London: Tavistock Publications.

WINNICOTT, D. W. (1957) *The Child and the Outside World*, London: Tavistock Publications.

WOMEN'S GROUP ON PUBLIC WELFARE (1948) *The Neglected Child and His Family*, London: Oxford University Press.

WORLD HEALTH ORGANISATION (1962) 'Deprivation of Maternal Care; a reassessment of its effects', *Public Health Papers*, 14, Geneva: W.H.O.

WYNNE, M. (1964) *Fatherless Families*, London: Michael Joseph.

YOUNG, P., WARHAM, J. & PETTES, D. (1967) *Administration and Staff Supervision in the Child Care Service*, London: Association of Child Care Officers.

YOUNGHUSBAND, E. ed. (1965) *Social Work with Families*, London: Allen & Unwin.

YELLOLY, M. (1966) 'Adoption and the Natural Mother,' *Case Conference*, Vol. XIII No. 8, Dec. 1966.


*Autobiographical*

HITCHMAN, J. (1960) *King of the Barbareens*, London: Putnam & Co.

HOLMES, G. V. (1948) *The Likes of Us*, London: Frederick Muller.

SINCLAIR, L. (1956) *The Bridgeburn Days*, London: Gollancz.

THOMAS, L. (1964) *This Time Next Week*, London: Constable & Co.

T - #0231 - 101024 - C0 - 198/129/7 [9] - CB - 9781032440699 - Gloss Lamination